Better
Health

ABOUT THE AUTHORS

Kirsten Hartvig ND, MRN, Dip. Phyt. MNIMH, is a registered naturopath, a medical herbalist, and an experienced international lecturer on the art of living and healing naturally. Before studying herbalism and naturopathy, she trained as a psychotherapist. After several years working in conventional consultation settings (during which time she also taught nutrition and dietetics at the European School of Osteopathy), she left practice to run residential healing retreats and to give courses and public lectures on herbal medicine and healthy eating in Britain, Denmark and France. She has written six books, most recently, *Eat for Immunity*. Her main interest is to help people take charge of their own health using widely available foods, herbs and simple naturopathic techniques.

Dr Nic Rowley read medicine at Trinity College, Cambridge and completed his clinical training in London. He is also qualified in acupuncture. He was Vice Principal at the European School of Osteopathy, and has worked as a holistic physician in multi-disciplinary practices in Kent and West Sussex. Nic is the author of *Basic Clinical Service*, *Describing a Rose with a Ruler* – a standard reference for students of complementary medicine – and *Hands On, A Manual of Clinical Skills*. He has also collaborated with Kirsten Hartvig on four other books – *Energy Foods*, *Energy Drinks*, *The Detox Book* and *You Are What You Eat*.

Nic and Kirsten together run a retreat in France.

10 Days
to
Better
Health

A step-by-step programme to
restore good health and vitality

KIRSTEN HARTVIG ND &
DR NIC ROWLEY

PIATKUS

This book is dedicated with
love and thanks to
Anna Clemence Mews

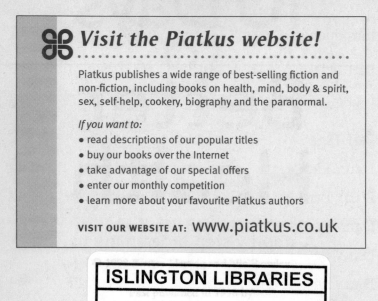

ꗠ Visit the Piatkus website!

Piatkus publishes a wide range of best-selling fiction and
non-fiction, including books on health, mind, body & spirit,
sex, self-help, cookery, biography and the paranormal.

If you want to:
- read descriptions of our popular titles
- buy our books over the Internet
- take advantage of our special offers
- enter our monthly competition
- learn more about your favourite Piatkus authors

VISIT OUR WEBSITE AT: www.piatkus.co.uk

The moral right of the authors has been asserted

A catalogue record for this book is available from the British Library

ISBN 0–7499–2438–1

Designed by Paul Saunders
Diagrams by Rodney Paull

Typeset by Phoenix Photosetting, Chatham, Kent
Printed and bound in Great Britain by
Mackays Ltd, Chatham, Kent

CONTENTS

ACKNOWLEDGEMENTS

We would like to express our love and gratitude to all those who have spent time on retreat with us over the past few years, and who have taught us so much about health and self-healing. In particular we would like to thank Jackie Young, Birgitte Haldbo, Katinka Thielemans, Joyce Thomas, Linda Wilkinson, Richard Wilkinson, Lilly Jensen, Anna Mews, Ernst Frederiksen, Peter Firebrace, Tara Lucis Firebrace, Jennifer Maughan, Lynne Misseldine, Rob Ward and Heather Rocklin for all their kindness, help and encouragement.

INTRODUCTION

※

Ten Days To Better Health is a step-by-step guide to self-healing. It uses simple, natural, low-cost methods, and includes a variety of powerful techniques to help relieve stress and increase vitality. It can be used in any home, any time and by virtually everyone. It doesn't involve taking time off work, seeing therapists, or using costly supplements. It is about living in the present, taking personal responsibility for health and improving quality of life right now.

Each day for ten days you will follow a Daily Programme Guide designed to help you introduce better nutrition, proper rest and gentle exercise into your normal routine, and to create a healthier balance between work, rest and play in your life. The elements of these Guides are very simple, and include plenty of sleep, quiet times, daily walks and the use of herbs and oils to reduce stress, improve energy levels and aid digestion. You will learn to prepare tasty, satisfying, healthy meals, and will carry out short Health Workshops in which you will experience different ways of awakening your own self-healing power. You will go through a process of change and transformation which unfolds over the ten days, a journey through the process of healing.

Part One, A Time for Healing, explains the naturopathic principles on which the programme is based and describes the techniques you will be using. Part Two, Preparation, guides you through the process of creating a healing environment, and contains advice on how to tailor the programme to your own particular situation. The Daily Programme Guides in Part Three set out the practical programme in a clear and consistent format. Each Guide contains all the information you will need for each day and includes detailed recipes and notes on the healing properties of the foods, herbs, spices and oils used. You won't have to look elsewhere in the book (or in other books) to follow the programme successfully. Recipes are quick and easy to prepare and are chosen to give you maximum health benefit for minimum cost. The Health Workshops are presented in clear, non-technical language and will allow you to get a real feel for various healing techniques, but without spending ages reading or preparing. The Conclusion includes hints and tips on incorporating naturopathic methods into your daily life once you have finished the programme, and is followed by an appendix containing further examples of the use of essential oils, water, fasting and ceremony as part of a self-help strategy for continuing health. The book ends with some suggestions for further reading and a list of useful addresses.

There are many ways of encouraging health, and the growth in the number of therapies available to treat any given illness is a remarkable aspect of life in the late twentieth century. When we saw patients in a conventional consultation setting, we ourselves used to use acupuncture, aromatherapy, Bach remedies, counselling, dietary therapy, herbal medicine, homeopathy, hydrotherapy and psychotherapy alongside and in place of conventional medicine. Despite the undoubted value of these and many other types of medical intervention, however, seeing patients in this way seemed to us somehow incomplete – a sort of 'once a week holism' which placed the emphasis on the remedy or treatment rather than on the self-healing power of the individual.

Time and again we found ourselves in the situation of using a daily medicine or weekly therapy to battle with 24-hour-a-day problems caused by a lack of the basic necessities of health – good sleep, good nutrition, good exercise and good environment – and we realized that it is impossible to tell how ill someone really is until these basics are sorted out. Rest, food, activity and surroundings affect our physical, mental, emotional, spiritual and healing abilities in the most profound way (a fact known since ancient times and confirmed by modern science), and to use any medical intervention without first paying attention to the basics is like lighting a candle in the wind.

In an attempt to put our practice where our mouth was, so to speak, we started having people come to stay with us, offering them a simple mix of relaxation, good food, time outdoors and in the garden, gentle activity, therapeutic baths, silence, music, song, laughter and space. Instead of being therapists, we became observers of people discovering their own self-healing capacity through simple means and learning through experience new skills that helped them stay healthy. We saw that the real causes of disease are more easily discovered in a safe and restful environment, and that everyone knows deep inside what makes them ill and what makes them better.

As our work with retreat continued and developed, we realized that the process of healing evolves through distinct phases and the more we observed, the more we realized that a healing environment could be created in any home by anyone – as long as they had the necessary information. The capacity for self-healing is a natural gift given to every one of us; health is not the property of the medical elite.

Following the programme set out in this book will enable you to experience the healing power of retreat for yourself and will introduce you to a wide range of powerful healing techniques. It will help you rid your body and mind of accumulated waste and detoxify your system of the chemical and emotional rubbish that modern life may have dumped on you. If you are basically healthy, it will improve your energy levels and leave you feeling lighter, calmer and more focused. If you are ill, it will provide a sure foundation for true healing and provide you with a whole battery of self-help skills. Whatever your state of health, it will rest, soothe and relax your body, mind and spirit, and give you the chance you have been promising yourself to take some time to sort yourself out. It will help you to establish a more healthy life-style by restoring your link with the healing power of nature.

Human beings are all the same and the thing that makes them all the same is that they are all different. Thus, healing is always a unique and personal matter and no two people following a self-help programme will have exactly the same experience. But the power to get healthy and stay healthy exists within you and the key to releasing it is to realize that just because you can't solve all your problems doesn't mean that you can't solve some of them. And the more you solve, the easier it becomes to solve the rest.

A man came on retreat complaining of a skin problem that would not go away. It emerged that his wife had recently died of cancer after a long and painful illness during which he had looked after her at home with little help or support. Two years before her cancer was diagnosed, their son had committed suicide. Which medical treatment could heal his bleeding heart and cure his loneliness? Soothing creams eased his painful itching skin a little but, while they enabled him to deal with his stress a bit better, they couldn't solve the problem of what had happened and what to do with the rest of his life. Healing may start in the consultation room but the real work is done at home and has as much to do with changing attitude and life-style as with taking medicines and remedies. After a few days of rest, quiet, and a healthy diet, he began to take a new interest in himself and in life in general. As he became more aware of his self-healing ability, his view of life and death changed and his skin got better. By applying simple naturopathic principles, he was able to heal his skin and his heart.

Ten Days To Better Health will show you how to put naturopathic health principles into daily practice by using water, food, herbs and rest to restore health and vitality. It is about doing simple things well instead of reading about complicated things and never quite getting around to doing them. It will help you keep your balance on the see-saw of life by getting in touch with your own self-healing power.

Part One

A TIME FOR HEALING

※

We live today in a world of extremes, a world in which many of us struggle to maintain health and peace of mind. The pressures of modern life encourage us to act in ways that make us ill, and the increasing medicalization of society is sapping our confidence in our own self-healing abilities. Many of us are aware that it is important to have a healthy life-style, but most of us don't live healthily because changing our life-style seems impractical. Our education and the scientific climate of our times have convinced us that change has to be major if it is to be worthwhile, and that science and technology have a monopoly on power. Since the Industrial Revolution, machines have become more powerful, weapons more deadly and medicines ever stronger, while individuals have been weakened by having to rely on energy sources controlled by huge multinational corporations.

This is a book about individual power, about discovering within yourself the source of energy from which everything on Earth draws its strength – nature. Without earth, water, air and sunlight and the natural resources they create, there would be no life, no society, and no economic systems. All the technological advances that underpin modern life owe their existence to the energy and materials supplied by nature. In recognizing the natural forces within you, you can plug yourself into the system which *produces* the energy on which the world depends, and use this energy to be healthy.

To become skilled at using your in-built energy supply, however, you have to start looking inside yourself for answers. You have to realize that what happens tomorrow is a direct and inevitable consequence of what you do today, and that doing small things well is infinitely more effective than persistently avoiding doing big things; as a Chinese sage once said, 'all difficult things in the world start from the easy, all great things in the world start from the small'. At the same time, you have to learn to deal with things from where you are instead of not dealing with them because you are not where you want to be. Journeys of a thousand miles really do start from the spot under your feet. The journey to health through self-healing is not always fast, but with every step your confidence in your inner strength will grow and you will learn not to fear moving forward slowly, only not moving at all.

Natural Philosophy of Health

We are a part of nature and can learn much about the the process of self-healing by observing how nature works. Consider the procession of the seasons which encourages plants to grow from seed to bloom. Winter may seem like a period of darkness and cold, but its starkness also reveals the true landscape as trees lose their leaves and the undergrowth dies back. It is a time for removing dead wood, for pruning and clearing and for letting go of what has not been used while the land and its creatures rest. Though winter seems to be a time of little action and slow movement, day by day the light is returning and, with the emergence of spring, the impulse to clean, repair and renew asserts itself. The pace of life quickens and the appearance of first buds and new shoots heralds flowers and blossoms to come.

As the sun climbs higher in the sky, the brightness of spring merges imperceptibly into the deep warmth of summer when growth and diversity flourish, driven by an unstoppable inner momentum and nurtured by soft summer rain. Then, all of a sudden, all is ripe for harvest and the Earth is hushed in momentary wonder before the rush of cutting and picking that allows this miracle of abundance to be shared. Through mellow autumn the harvest is sorted and stored, and fuel is laid in for another period of rest and rejuvenation. The seeds that have fallen to earth are gently covered by leaves that moments ago captured the sunlight, and which will now return their substance back to the soil to nurture new life and new harvests. And suddenly it is winter once more, black branches outlined in white against a darkening sky.

So it is with self-healing. The first step is to see clearly where you are, to cut down and clear that which is no longer helpful in your life and to prune anything which has become overgrown. Next, you have to acknowledge your need for rest so that you can gather the energy that will fuel repair and regeneration. As the first signs of healing emerge, they need tending like delicate shoots in spring while you clean and tidy your mental and physical environment to provide maximum opportunity for future growth. As healing becomes established, you must make sure that you remain properly fed and watered during the period of rapid change so that the harvest of health is sure and abundant. And, as you gather your crop of wellbeing and plant the seeds of change that will determine your course over the next year, you should remember to lay up reserves against the exertions of new challenges and, in your dealings with others, be mindful of the fact that no harvest is complete until it is shared.

These ideas form the basis of naturopathy, a natural philosophy of health that provides the foundation for all traditional systems of medicine. Naturopathy sees health as a natural state and regards disease as nature's way of restoring health when an individual is out of balance with their environment. It recognizes that all healing is ultimately dependent on nature – the surgeon may set the bone but it is the body that actually mends the break. It suggests that the aim of all treatment should be to create the best possible circumstances for the body to heal itself, while avoiding anything that may do harm. It acknowledges the existence of a life-force which fuels our biological vehicle, and sees body, mind, emotion and spirit as interwoven strands in the fabric of life. It emphasizes the responsibility of each individual to create conditions favouring health.

In practical terms, naturopathy is about doing whatever you are doing now as well as possible, because it's what you do now that ultimately determines what happens to you next. In other words, do good now and good will happen. When it comes to health, this means paying attention to the basics – rest, play, nutrition, activity and community – before doing anything else. If we don't sleep, laugh, eat, drink, move and relate to others, we get ill.

The Road to Illness

We live in a society that tends to judge the value of individuals by their financial status, a fact which causes many people to sacrifice their health in the pursuit of wealth. We have also come to believe that our capacity to perform is limited only by the strength of our desire to achieve, and often act as if the body was an unlimited natural resource (in much the same way that we used to regard coal, oil and natural gas as unlimited sources of fuel). As a result, many of us have depleted our energy reserves so much that we have lost our capacity for self-healing, and this has made us increasingly dependent on powerful medical interventions to keep us going.

The diagram opposite shows how achievement and pressure are related in most people's lives, and illustrates three very important things. First, that if we have no incentive to do very much then we don't actually achieve very much; second, that increasing pressure to achieve tends to produce increased achievement, at least for a time; and third that if the pressure to perform gets too much, the ability to achieve inevitably decreases. When we perform better and achieve more (by working longer hours, taking on new responsibilities, being more productive) we get rewarded (with more prestige, more money, nicer things, more respect), and this convinces us that doing more brings us more of the things that we want. So we put even stronger pressure on ourselves to perform, in order to achieve the things we believe would free us from the pressures that others put on us. We act as if the line on our achievement graph will go on climbing if we can just push that bit harder, and think that tomorrow's rewards will compensate for today's worry.

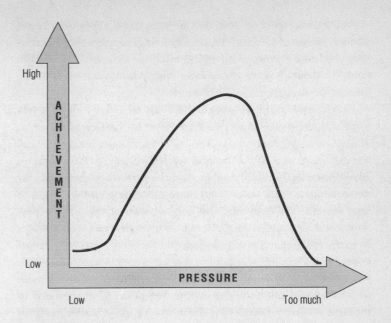

The reality is, however, that your ability to go on responding to pressure by increasing your level of performance is limited by your capacity to stay *healthy* in the face of increased pressure. Whether you like it or not, it is a biological fact that too much stress for too long will make you ill, and if you want to be healthy you have to understand that your inner energy store is a finite and precious resource to be used wisely when necessary, conserved where possible, and restocked at regular intervals.

In fact, the road to illness or breakdown in a person's life usually follows a fixed path, but the pattern is so common and the time scale so long that we often fail to notice it. As our lives unfold from youth to early adulthood, the external pressures that motivate us to perform – the need to earn enough to pay our bills, wanting promotion, letters from bank managers, the demands of parents, partners and friends – gradually increase, and our lives become fuller and busier. If tiredness, stress or worry intrude on our ambitions, society provides a range of pick-me-ups and calm-me-downs (tea, coffee, caffeine-packed soft drinks, cigarettes, chocolate, sugar, alcohol, recreational drugs) to keep us going, supplemented as necessary by 'minor' medical interventions. If we're lucky, illnesses also tend to be minor as we experiment with pushing ourselves to the limit in the struggle to 'make it' in life.

At a certain point, however, the battle to achieve or maintain material success – or simply to keep going in the face of failure or disillusionment – starts to take a toll. Sleep no longer brings rest, and we start each new day as tired as we left yesterday. Relationships grow brittle and unsatisfying, performance at work drops off, illnesses become more serious and more demanding and we begin to long for rest. Paradoxically, the help on offer at this stage – prescription drugs, counselling, alternative therapies, etc. – encourages us in the belief that if we could just find the right remedy, then we could go on coping. Each intervention brings some measure of relief, but we tend to use any energy regained to go on doing more of what caused our problems in the first place. Our approach to problem solving becomes 'if it doesn't work, do it harder', and we find it increasingly difficult to hear our inner voice saying 'if it doesn't work, do something else'.

The fact is, if what you are doing is tending to bring exhaustion, illness and disintegration into your life, things will inevitably get worse if you keep on doing it. But if you change what you do and start treating the basics of life as basic, you will become healthier and ensure that today's achievements form the foundation of a sustainable future. If you are tired, you need to rest; if you are damaged, you need time to heal. No one would think of running a marathon with a broken leg, so why persist in trying to run your life beyond the limits of your physical, mental and emotional endurance?

The Road to Health

There is an expression in computing 'rubbish in, rubbish out', which means that although computers are incredibly quick at doing what you tell them to do, if what you tell them to do is rubbish then the answers they come up with are also rubbish. The same is true of bodies. A body that learns to be healthy knows how to stay healthy, but a body under constant stress almost invariably becomes ill.

The human body is a remarkable self-regulating system, capable of providing a constant and congenial internal environment for you to live in despite the ever-changing world outside. Once it has learned what is expected of it, it can carry out a huge number of tasks on your behalf without ever pausing to ask for instructions. It keeps your temperature constant, adjusts your chemistry and control systems according to circumstances, and has a breathtaking repertoire of automatic skills which help you navigate through the day. Think of what a newborn baby can't do, and then think what you can do. From using a fork to driving a car, your body's ability to carry out tasks automatically that it learned previously by repetition is fundamental to your life, your ability to think, and to your free will.

In fact, the body could be described as a super-sophisticated learning-by-doing machine. Walking, eating, talking, riding a bike, driving a car, singing, playing the piano, catching a ball, kicking a football, chopping wood, carrying a glass of water without spilling it – the body learns how to do these things by doing them, and how it learns things first is how it goes on doing them unless you teach it to do something else. Everyone who has learned to drive and then tries driving a different car understands this. For some miles it is hard to operate the clutch, brake and accelerator smoothly, but go on doing it for long enough and the body learns. In all activity, the subconscious mind organizes the complex patterns of movement and response that enable you to do simple things like drink a cup of tea without pausing to remember how it's done. Your daily life depends to a large extent on the ability of your subconscious-controlled body to do things without you having to think about them.

Just as a muscle grows strong by repetition of its movement, the subconscious grows efficient by repeated experience, so if you want to change anything in your life you have to actually do something new, and keep on doing it long enough for your subconscious to learn how it's done. Whatever you think consciously will make absolutely no difference to your behaviour unless what you think leads to action, experience and new learning. What we call knowledge is often based on other people's experiences, and is very little use in changing anything unless it inspires us to act. We may know it's time to get a new battery, but it's the experience of it going flat that changes knowledge into action.

The point is that although you may want to be healthier, happier, calmer, more relaxed and more energetic, if you are currently not any of these things it is because your subconscious has learned habits that tend to make you unhealthy, sad, agitated, tense and lethargic. To remedy the situation, you have to re-programme the system by having a new range of experiences which teach your body-mind to let you feel how you actually want to feel. Once you have understood that doing certain things makes you feel better, you can learn how to do those things automatically by doing them a lot to start with. Like the basic living skills that a child learns (drinking, eating, walking, talking, bowel and bladder control and dressing), basic health skills become automatic once you have learned them, but take some patience and a lot of repetition early on.

About the Programme

During the course of *Ten Days To Better Health* you will try out a dozen different simple natural healing techniques, and will follow an appetizing naturopathic diet. You will spend some time each day outdoors and will have regular quiet times for relaxation and reflection. Once the programme is underway you will keep a diary of your dreams and will also do some simple observation exercises designed to focus attention on particular aspects of the environment relevant to the theme of each day. The emphasis throughout is on experiencing things rather than reading about them, so don't be surprised if you are asked sometimes to do things without much explanation about *why* you should do them. Like one brushstroke in a painting or one note in a tune, individual elements of the programme may have little significance by themselves, but together they build into a pattern of experience that encourages the process of healing. The following descriptions should help you get a feel for the gentle methods used in *Ten Days To Better Health*.

Throughout the ten days of the programme, you will be eating according to the principles of *naturopathic nutrition*, a fresh approach to healthy eating based on age-old knowledge. Founded on the idea that you are what you eat, it is a way of making any diet healthy using cheap, widely available foods and without using vitamin or mineral supplements. By eating more of what is good for you instead of worrying about what is bad for you, you will eat more complex carbohydrates, fibre, vitamins and minerals and less fat and sugar. By filling your stomach with healthy food, you will leave less room for the unhealthy. To encourage the process of cleansing and detoxification, the programme menus become increasingly simple over the first few days so that on the fifth day you eat only fruit. From then until day ten, the meals become progressively more substantial. *Ten Days To Better Health* is NOT a weight loss programme or an exercise in self-denial. You may or may not lose a couple of pounds, depending on your constitution, but the object of the diet is to support and nourish your body through a time of change and healing.

Throughout the programme you will be introduced to a variety of natural healing techniques:

• **Herbalism** is the ancient understanding of the healing properties of plants which forms a part of most traditional systems of healing and medicine. Its remedies are safe, cheap and widely available, and many common plants and weeds can be used as effective medicines. Herbalism in its simplest form uses fresh or dried herbs to make pleasant tasting teas (and to flavour healthy recipes) as a way of encouraging and supporting the body to heal itself. Unlike many pharmaceutical remedies, herbs are generally free of harmful side-effects and contain important vitamins and minerals in addition to medicinal substances. They can therefore make a significant contribution to the nutritional quality of any diet.

• **Aromatherapy** is the use of natural oils extracted from plants to restore or enhance health and general wellbeing. Essential oils can be used in massage, baths, oils burners, inhalations, compresses, perfumes and even cooking to relax and invigorate the body, mind and spirit, and can be powerful aids to healing and stress management. Though aromatherapy oils are concentrated, sometimes expensive substances, it needs only small amounts to produce a beneficial effect.

• **Hydrotherapy** is the art of using water to treat illness and improve health and is a central feature of all nature-cure and health-spa regimes. Hot and cold baths of all types (including footbaths and sitz-baths), showers, wraps, steam inhalations and the drinking of mineral waters are all proven ways of using nature to nurture the body, and most hydrotherapy techniques can be used by anyone with access to a tap and a bath-tub.

• **Stretching** is something we all do naturally from time to time, and cats and dogs have developed it into a fine art. Many ancient exercise methods such as Tai Chi, Qi Gong and Yoga are based on the systematic stretching of different muscle groups around the body, and modern research has shown that regular stretching is a powerful way of maintaining the health of bones and the mobility of joints. Stretching routines can be adapted to suit any age or body type, take a minimum of space and time and require no special equipment to be effective.

• **Breathing** is the fundamental activity of life. Without food we can survive for weeks, without water for days, but without air entering our lungs we die within minutes. Since getting fresh oxygen into our bodies and waste carbon dioxide out is the basis of every thought, movement and activity we perform, it is commonsense to make sure that we learn how to breathe as effectively and efficiently as possible. Since breathing is for the most part an unconscious activity, most of us never give a second thought to how we are breathing and, as a result, many of us breathe inefficiently. Simple exercises can help you make the most of the air you breathe and make you feel brighter, more energetic and very much more relaxed. They can help improve the way you speak, sing, move and sleep and, like stretching, require nothing except a bit of enthusiasm, and a determination to learn.

• **Massage** can be used for relaxation and also to treat various aches, pains and injuries, but self-massage is less well known. In some oriental cultures, self-massage techniques to relieve tension and promote health are handed down in families and even taught in schools. Self-massage is quick to learn, easy to do and can even be done without taking off your clothes. The system used in *Ten Days To Better Health* is based on Chinese and Japanese methods and can be used anytime to relax muscular tension and stimulate the flow of energy around the body.

• **Relaxation** is a dying art in late twentieth-century society; it is slowly being replaced by leisure activities that require thought and activity and which, in some cases, are positively stimulating (such as watching TV and playing computer games). True relaxation is a state of rest of body, mind and emotions and, like any art, takes some practice to master. All healing traditions stress the importance of relaxation in the maintenance of health, and there are nowadays a wide variety of relaxation methods on offer from therapists and self-help books. The method introduced in *Ten Days To Better Health* is based on a yoga technique which is simple, effective and easy to use. It requires no tapes or other aids and can be used whenever the pressure of life starts to get too much.

• **Self-audit.** The *Concise Oxford Dictionary* defines 'audit' as a 'searching examination' and, at some point in the process of self-healing, a period of self-audit – an examination of the self – is always necessary. This is because most of us carry around a suitcase full of unresolved worries and tensions that have their roots in our past experiences and which have a powerful influence on our behaviour and our health. The self-audit workshop of *Ten Days To Better Health* is a chance to open the suitcase of memories, look at what's inside and take out anything in there that is unnecessary in order to make your journey through life a little easier. It involves remembering and reviewing key moments in your personal history, and can be an important step on the path towards answering the question 'Who am I?'

• **Autosuggestion** is a powerful self-healing method based on a simple idea – if your mind is capable of letting you walk, eat, wash, write, drive a car and carry out a whole range of complex tasks without you having to think about how they're done, it must also be capable of making and keeping you healthy once it knows how. This old concept is fully supported by modern science which now rejects the idea that the mind and body are separate. A mind/body split may seem common-sensical, but only if you make the mistake of thinking that your mind consists only of what you know you are thinking. In fact, your mind is constantly initiating, monitoring and controlling a whole range of automatic activities which enable you to do what you want to do, and is intimately involved with your fundamental body processes. Everyone knows the feeling in the pit of the stomach (and the pounding in the chest) that accompanies a shock or surprise, and this is just one of countless examples of the mind and body acting as one. If what you think can change your adrenaline level, alter your blood pressure, adjust your hormonal secretions and influence your immune system, then you can use what you think to help your body work better. Once you have understood this, you can also use your mind to calm and control your emotions. All you have to realize is that if you want your subconscious mind to do something for you, you have to tell it – and keep on telling it until it understands. Above all, taking control of what your mind learns and does helps you to resist the constantly repeated messages of the modern world which do so much for the profit of multinational corporations and so little for individual peace of mind – go there, buy this, look like that, eat the other, drink more, smoke anyway; and so on, countless times each day. Advertising and sales people understand clearly that the mind and body work as one, but old-fashioned science has convinced many of us that they are separate, and this often prevents us from taking control of our lives. In *Ten Days To Better Health*, autosuggestion is used as a way of *you* deciding what you do, how you feel and what you think.

• **Meditation** conjures up different images in different people. To some it suggests relaxation, to others religion and prayer, but to many it also carries connotations of weirdness, candles, cults and escapist navel-gazing. Nevertheless, nearly everyone has had experience of meditation – even if they don't recognize it as such – because everyone has some way of finding a bit of mental calm amid the clamour of life. Going for a walk, squinting at a sun-sparkled sea, listening to music, sewing, gardening, idly watching the world go by – these, and many other simple pastimes, absorb our thoughts, quieten our minds and take us out of ourselves and so give us the experience of inner silence that is the essence of meditation. The point of learning to meditate in a structured way is that it allows you to recreate those precious moments of calm whenever and wherever you need or want to. This in turn helps to improve creativity and concentration, and ensures that you get the most from your available energy. The meditation method described in *Ten Days To Better Health* is not based on any particular philosophy or religion, and poses no challenge to other systems you may already know.

• **Music and dance** have always played a role in healing, but the development of modern mass-media has meant that few people now have the daily experience of dancing or making music for themselves. On the other hand, the current resurgence of interest in line dancing and circle dancing, and the perennial strength of local choirs, choral societies and music groups bear witness to the importance of music and movement as basic human needs. The penultimate workshop in *Ten Days To Better Health* is a reminder that we all have a capacity for music and rhythm, and can all feel better for singing and dancing once in a while.

• **Ceremony.** If you follow a religion, the chances are that one of the things that drew you to it in the first place was the type of ceremony and ritual it used. Even if you have no interest in religion, ceremony will still play an important role in your life since so much of society is organized along ceremonial lines. As well as obvious examples (like weddings and state occasions), job interviews, business meetings, parties, passing out parades, prize givings and school assemblies all embody the spirit of ceremony. Many daily tasks, from getting ready for work each morning to washing the car on a Sunday afternoon, are also performed in a ritual way. A stranger from another planet would come to the conclusion that ceremony and ritual were a basic part of normal human behaviour used to mark important moments and confer rites of passage. The last workshop in *Ten Days To Better Health* encourages you to design your own ceremony to mark the completion of the ten days, and to acknowledge the effort you have made.

The Spiritual Aspect

Naturopathy is based on the idea that health is a state of balance between our physical, emotional, mental and spiritual aspects, and *Ten Days To Better Health* involves paying attention to all these qualities of self. The programme does not seek to put forward a particular view of spirituality, however, and does not support a sectarian view of religion. Just as nature is life clothed in a million costumes, spirituality in human experience takes many forms. Nevertheless, the qualities that most of us would associate with spirituality – kindness, compassion, goodness and service – are welcome visitors whatever our personal belief system, and are the foundation of all true healing. There is no true health without love.

Cautions, Side-Effects and Special Needs

Ten Days To Better Health is a gentle and progressive programme designed to solve problems, not create them. It can be used by nearly everyone, although it is not intended for people suffering from serious acute illness or for young people under the age of eighteen, and we would not recommend following it during pregnancy and while breast feeding.

The programme will not interfere with any medication you may be taking and you should certainly not stop taking any prescribed drugs without first seeking the advice of the practitioner who prescribed them. If you are being treated for diabetes, you should be aware that your calorie intake may well be lower than normal during the middle days of the programme, and you should discuss the implications of this with your medical adviser before starting. Use your common-sense when it comes to doing the stretching exercises, avoiding strain and pain and limiting any movements likely to exacerbate pre-existing injury or weakness.

The programme is extremely unlikely to produce any unpleasant or serious side-effects, but you may notice that withdrawal from stimulants and relaxants like tea, coffee, alcohol and smoking makes you feel more edgy, head-achey, lethargic and short-tempered than usual for the first few days. The increase in fruit and vegetable intake may also make your bowels a bit loose, and the extra fibre may cause wind. Such symptoms soon pass, however, and are not a cause for concern. If you have skin that is particularly prone to allergic reactions, it may be wise to check your sensitivity to the various essential oils by rubbing a little diluted oil on to a small patch of skin on your forearm, the night before using it for the next day's bath or massage. As always, if you have any particular concerns or worries, you should seek advice from your doctor or, if he or she should feel unable to offer advice, from a registered naturopath.

Above all, remember that *Ten Days To Better Health* is not a 'treatment' for any particular condition or disease. It is a strategy to help you maximize your self-healing potential, a way of learning to be healthy by doing things that are healthy. The programme offers a simple way of applying naturopathic principles to daily life and uses methods as old as the human race adapted to a modern context. Follow it, and you will be healthier, calmer, more energetic and better nourished. You will develop a better understanding of health and disease, and will learn self-help skills which you can use to reduce stress and relieve illness. By putting goodness into your life, you will get health out of it.

Part Two

PREPARATION

❧

This part of the book is about creating a healing environment in your home, and the sorting out and deck-clearing that is necessary to get the most out of *Ten Days To Better Health*. It contains a detailed shopping list to make your preparation easier, and also a short life-style questionnaire which you can use to review your current situation.

Creating a Healing Environment

Many people dream of having a relaxing break in a health spa where they can eat healthily, rest, relax, 'take the waters' and generally feel pampered and cosseted. For most of us, however, work and family life plus the cost of such establishments make such dreams impossible; even proper holidays are luxuries often hard to afford.

Ironically, a fly on the wall at a health spa would see that the elements that make up expensive 'cures' are, in themselves, very simple and very cheap. Naturopathy is first and foremost a way of promoting health for all, based on things that nature gives for free – water, air, sunlight, sleep, movement, touch and wayside weeds – and can be used by anyone with a desire to improve their health. What the health spas have that most of the rest of us don't is information on how to use 'nature's healers' effectively, and the purpose of this book is to make such information available to you.

It may seem far fetched to say that you can create a mini-health spa in your own home, but with a little bit of effort and some preparation you can do just that. What is more, choosing to turn your home into a healing environment instead of wishing for a break somewhere else has many advantages. Home is familiar and hopefully safe. It doesn't involve costly or difficult travel or the need to get used to new surroundings. Using it as a place to get well is no more expensive than just living there in the first place, and any improvement in the home environment and in your state of health and vitality will also benefit others who share your home. Though the 'getting away from it all' experience may appear to be missing, introducing a new way of living for ten days in itself produces the change that is as good as a rest. Even the most well-known objects, people and places look different through fresh eyes. Best of all, there is no last-minute packing flurry or end-of-holiday blues to contend with. You will have learnt how to feel better in your own home on your own terms, and anything you discover during the programme that makes you feel good you can carry on doing afterwards.

In practical terms, creating a healing environment involves dealing with six things: time, space, people, backlogs, intrusions and habits.

Time

You should aim to start *Ten Days To Better Health* on a Wednesday, since days four and five work best when they fall on a weekend. The fact that the programme will end on a Friday evening is also helpful since you will then have a weekend to reflect on your experiences. Although the programme does not involve taking time off work or stopping your normal daily activities, you should make sure that you have no social or travel commitments during the ten days.

It is crucial that once you start the programme, you finish it, and it should only be interrupted in exceptional circumstances. Awakening your own self-healing ability is a powerful experience and it can be challenging to spend so much time and effort attending to your self and your own needs. Change requires changing, and there may be moments during the ten days when you feel that you can't be bothered to carry on. To give up at such a moment wastes the time and effort you put into getting started and means that you will never find out what would have happened if you had continued. Things only happen for the first time once.

Perhaps the main difference between *Ten Days To Better Health* and ten days at a health spa or on 'retreat' is that there is nobody except you encouraging you forward, but discovering your inner resources using your own inner strength is an intensely rewarding experience and definitely worth the effort involved.

Space

The programme requires two things in terms of space: first, a small area which can be your quiet, private space at any time during the ten days and second, a reasonably warm bathroom (with bath or shower). Spare bedrooms or tidied up boxrooms are potentially ideal quiet spaces, as long as they have room for a bed or a mattress and a chair, and are warm (or can be warmed up quickly). Other possibilities include your bedroom (after negotiations with your partner if necessary), garden sheds and summerhouses (depending on the weather!)

Try and make your quiet space as pleasant as you can, using things you already have around the house and covering up any eyesores with nice bits of material or sheets. An upright chair, a warm blanket, and a bed with a couple of cushions or pillows are the main things you will need in the room, although a small table or shelf may also be useful. If you don't have a spare bed or mattress, a large soft mat or blanket on the floor will do just as well. The lighting should be as gentle as possible, perhaps using candles or nightlights to create a cosy atmosphere, and you should arrange a few things around the room that you feel are special to you in some way, or that you find particularly beautiful (such as fresh flowers, plants, ornaments, or pictures). It helps if the room is not too cluttered, though.

If you are able to make your quiet space in a separate room, it is best to ask anyone who shares your house not to go into it for the ten days. If you have to use your bedroom as your quiet space and you share the room with a partner, you should negotiate as much private time in there as possible and keep one part of the room as your 'private corner'.

People

Before starting the programme, it is important to enlist the support of any family, friends and work colleagues who are likely to be affected by your following it. You will need to explain to them that for ten days you will be getting up earlier, going to bed earlier, spending a bit of time each morning and evening on your own, going for a walk at lunchtime, eating a bit differently and spending a little more time in the bathroom. Depending on your particular situation, these changes may have no effect on anyone, or may need some negotiation to allow the programme to run smoothly for you. In particular, if you are the main care and meal provider in your home, you may need to agree some temporary new arrangements over cooking, housecare and childcare with your partner, close family or friends to make it possible for you to relax and enjoy the programme.

When negotiating a little more time and space for yourself for ten days, remember that if you were seriously ill, your family and friends would happily adapt and help out to make it possible for you to get better; so it must make even more sense for them to make a few adjustments for just a few days to help you get more healthy. Remember, the programme doesn't involve you going away or stopping doing most of what you normally do. Whatever your basic daily responsibilities to work or home, you will continue to carry them out. All that will change is the time you get up and go to bed, the food you will be eating and the fact that you will be taking half an hour in the morning, fifteen minutes at the end of the day, one hour in the evening and fifteen minutes before bedtime to be by yourself. You may also spend a few minutes more in the bathroom, either in the morning or evening. All the other elements of the programme can be fitted into your normal routine.

A little bit of flexibility and goodwill is therefore all that should be necessary from your family and friends and, should the ten days benefit you, you will be able to encourage, advise and support them to follow your example. If, on the other hand, partners and family find the small adjustments needed to support you during the programme are too much, this may well mean that you yourself have got into a habit of doing too much each day. Negotiations over *Ten Days To Better Health* can be a useful preliminary to more detailed discussions about the division of labour and responsibility within your home, so that everyone has the best chance to preserve their health and vitality in the long term.

Backlogs

Perhaps the most important thing you can do to maximize the benefits of following *Ten Days To Better Health* is to make a concerted effort beforehand to clear up the backlogs in your life. The letters you meant to write, the people you meant to phone, the things that have been niggling at you for the past few weeks – getting as many of these out of the way as possible can bring a surprising improvement in health, energy and peace of mind all by itself, and can be a first and powerful step on the road to self-healing. It doesn't matter if you can't clear everything up, but at least try and do the things you would do if you were going away for ten days. Even though you are not actually going away, the peace of mind that comes from getting more sorted out will greatly enhance the effects of the programme on your health and vitality.

Intrusions

Preparing for *Ten Days To Better Health* is also an opportunity to take stock of the things in your life you find stressful, and to see if there are any practical ways of dealing with them. During the ten days, you should avoid TV, radio, newspapers, internet surfing, computer games and using the telephone completely while you are at home/not working (if you were at a health farm or on holiday, you wouldn't find this too difficult), and also as far as is practical at work. The programme is an opportunity to attend to your own thoughts and ideas, and to reduce for a time the influence on your life of other people's concerns. As with a holiday, when the programme is over you will find that very little has actually changed when you 'come back', except for you! If you feel the need for extra entertainment during the programme, listen to music. The ability of gentle music to help the mind to relax and re-order itself is phenomenal, and can be a powerful aid to self-healing.

If you find the early morning sound of post falling on the mat at all stressful, make a deal with yourself not to open or even look through the mail until after lunch (or early evening if you go out to work). This will make the start of the day more relaxing and will ensure that you are in the best frame of mind to deal with any new tasks or information that the post may bring. Noise, cold, heat, air pollution, over-burdened roads and over-crowded, inefficient public transport are other stress factors which can be hard to avoid or alter. Being alert to any and every possibility to reduce the impact of these on your life – even by a small amount – may add up to a significant reduction in daily stress, however. Car sharing, a new route, a travel time altered by just five minutes – even wearing a different item of clothing – can make all the difference to the stress of an average day.

Perhaps the most important stress factors in life are the demands others put on us and the demands we put on ourselves. Children and parents, partners and friends, bosses and employees, ambition and conscience; all form a web of responsibilities and obligations in which we sometimes feel trapped. Finding a good balance between what we do for others, what others do for us and what we do for ourselves is one of life's major challenges. The bottom line is that the good you are able to do for others is founded on the good you do yourself. If what you are able to do for others depends entirely on what others have to do for you, there is no net benefit to anyone in the long run. If the good you do for others is founded on energy *you* generate by doing good to yourself, everyone gains.

Habits

Smoking, alcohol and stimulants like caffeine-containing drinks and beverages (tea, coffee, colas, etc.) are so much part of twentieth-century life that we barely give them a second thought. If we like their taste or depend on their effects, it is easy to ignore three facts:

1 Smoking is unquestionably bad for health and is the clear cause of several of the commonest major killing and disabling diseases in modern society.

2 Alcohol in all but the most moderate amounts is a dangerous, powerful and addictive drug responsible for millions of avoidable deaths and ruined lives each year.

3 Stimulant-containing drinks and beverages give you energy in the short term by making you use your energy quicker. If you don't have the energy to do something without a stimulant, you shouldn't do it at all if you want to avoid depleting your energy stores in the long term.

Whichever way you look at it, doing harm to your health can't do it good, so if you are doing the programme because you want to be more healthy, cutting out (or at least cutting down) on these three habits for a short time is a major step in the right direction. *Ten Days To Better Health* is a chance to give up all these habits for ten days.

Tailoring the Programme to Your Situation

In planning when to start *Ten Days To Better Health*, remember that the programme is a chance to use your energy for your own needs. You should therefore reduce your social commitments to a minimum and avoid difficult business meetings if possible. If you are feeling very run down – and particularly if you suffer from a chronic illness of some sort – you should consider taking some leave or time off work during the ten days to allow yourself maximum opportunity for rest and healing. Similarly, you might consider asking family and/or friends to give you additional help with childcare, or you might choose to follow the programme when partner, children or both are due to be away. If your home situation is difficult, you may even decide to take yourself off somewhere completely different for ten days (although it should be somewhere that you can still have a private space and cook for yourself).

It might also be helpful to follow the programme at the same time as a close friend or relative, if you feel this would make the preparation more fun or if you would value having someone to share the experience with. Whatever your individual circumstances, the object is to create a time and space in your life that gives you the best possible chance to complete the programme without interruption.

What You Will Need

Apart from yourself, a quiet space and a bathroom, the main things you need in order to follow *Ten Days To Better Health* are some dried herbs, some essential oils and the ingredients for the daily recipes. Most of the foods and some of the herb teas should be available at local grocery stores, although if you want to use organic produce you may have to contact the Soil Association (*see* Useful Addresses) to find the name of a local supplier. The less common herbs can sometimes be found in health-food stores. Essential oils can be bought in a variety of bodycare shops and most health-food stores these days.

To simplify your shopping, Neal's Yard Remedies will supply by mail order a special 'Ten Days To Better Health pack' containing the right amounts of all the herbs and oils required for the programme. Purchasing this pack will help to avoid waste and ensure that you get products of the highest quality at a reasonable cost (see Useful Addresses).

Apart from foods, herbs and oils, you will also need a tea strainer, some strips of old material, a candle holder and some candles or nightlights, a watch or clock, five coloured pens or crayons (red, yellow, green, blue and purple), and a largish notebook (with pen). If you don't have a bathtub, you will also need a large bowl or washtub for some of the hydrotherapy exercises.

Shopping Lists

Here is the full shopping list for the programme. If you have any of the herbs or oils already, so much the better; but try to collect all the herbs and oils you will need before starting the ten days. The food shopping-list is divided into four parts: non-perishable (to buy before starting the programme); fresh produce for Days 1 to 5; extra shopping (to be done on Day 4); fresh produce for Days 6 to 10.

Herbs and Oils

- A box of teabags – or 30 grams (1 ounce) of loose dried herb – of each of the following herbs: peppermint, fennel, thyme, chamomile, nettle, yarrow, vervain, St John's wort, and angelica.
- 2 mls (or the smallest available bottle) of each of the following essential oils: eucalyptus, marjoram, pine, lavender, rosemary, melissa, frankincense, sandalwood and rose.
- 15mls of maccrated calendula oil and 100mls of sweet almond oil to dilute the other oils.

Foods

The quantities listed below are per person. If some of the foods are not available in your area, feel free to choose alternatives.

Non-perishable (to buy before starting the programme)

300g/11oz dried apricots
350g/12½oz dried dates
100g/3½oz raisins
1 small packet dessicated coconut
150g/6oz shelled nuts and seeds (e.g., walnuts, hazelnuts, almonds, cashews, pine kernels, sesame seeds, sunflower seeds, melon seeds)
50g/2oz couscous grains
250g/9oz sugar-free muesli base
80g/3oz rolled oats
250g/9oz long-grain brown rice
50g/2oz wheat flour
1 small bottle maple syrup
1 small jar French mustard
1 small jar olives (optional)

1 packet vegetable stock cubes (free from monosodium glutamate)
1 small jar capers
1 medium jar tahini paste
250mls/9fl oz olive oil
120mls/5fl oz safflower oil
75mls/3fl oz walnut oil
100g/4oz tinned chick-peas (or 50g/2oz dried)
100g/4oz dried red lentils
2 litres/4pts unsweetened soya milk
1 small bottle soy sauce
1 small tin sweetcorn
dried herbs and spices: basil, bay leaf, cayenne (optional),
    cinnamon (optional), coriander seeds, cumin seeds, curry
    powder (optional), herbes de Provence, horseradish (optional),
    mint, oregano, paprika, thyme and tumeric.

If you are concerned about the quality of your local tap water, buy
ten large bottles of still mineral water to drink during the programme.

Fresh Produce for days 1 to 5

Vegetables:
1 avocado, 1 bunch fresh chives, 1 bunch fresh mint, 1 small bunch
coriander leaf, 1 small bunch fresh parsley, 2 beetroot, 1 small head
broccoli, 8 carrots, 1 parsnip, 1 courgette, 1 small celeriac, 1
medium bunch celery, 1 cucumber, 1 fennel, 1 iceberg lettuce,
60g/2oz mushrooms, 2 onions, 1 red onion, 1 large head garlic, 1
green pepper, 1 red pepper, 1 small bunch spring onions, 1 small
bunch radishes, 575g/1lb 5oz potatoes, 100g/4oz sorrel leaves
(optional), 100g/4oz spinach, 5 tomatoes, 60g/2oz bean sprouts,
225g/8oz mixed root vegetables, 1 bunch watercress (optional).

Fruits and berries:
2 lemons, 7 apples, 7 bananas, 1 orange, 1 grapefruit, 225g/8oz
grapes, 400g/14oz mixed fresh fruit/berries (e.g., apricots, peaches,
nectarines, plums, cherries, raspberries, strawberries, blackcurrants,
redcurrants), 2 apricots (optional).

Miscellaneous:

2 litres/4pts unsweetened fruit juice, 1l/2pts mixed vegetable juice

Extra Shopping for Day 5 (to be done on Day 4)

1 mango, 1 paw paw or 1 melon, 3 pears, 1 pineapple, 150g/5oz grapes, 500g/1lb 2oz mixed fresh fruit/berries (e.g., apricots, peaches, nectarines, plums, cherries, raspberries, strawberries, black-currants, redcurrants).

Fresh Produce for days 6 to 10

Vegetables:

3 avocados, 1 bunch fresh basil, 1 bunch fresh mint, 1 bunch water-cress (optional), 1 small bunch fresh parsley, 200g/7oz green beans, 4 large open mushrooms, 2 medium beetroot, 1 small head broc-coli, 1 small red cabbage, 4 carrots, 1 cauliflower, 1 courgette, 1 endive, 1 small piece fresh ginger, 1 small piece horseradish, 1 ice-berg lettuce, 150g/6oz mushrooms, 1 large onion (or 3 shallots), small bunch spring onions, 1 small bunch radishes, 500g/1lb 2oz potatoes, 150g/6oz spinach (or 100g/4oz frozen), 2 tomatoes.

Fruits and berries:

2 lemons, 7 apples, 5 bananas, 1 grapefruit, 1 kiwi fruit, 2 oranges, 100g/4oz grapes, 750g/1lb 10oz other mixed fruit/berries (e.g., apricots, peaches, nectarines, plums, cherries, raspberries, strawber-ries, blackcurrants, redcurrants).

Miscellaneous:

2 litres/4pts unsweetened fruit juice, 1 loaf bread, 1 carton soya yoghurt, 120g/4oz tofu.

Costs

Food shopping for *Ten Days To Better Health* should cost you no more than your normal diet (and, since you will not be consum-ing some of the more expensive foods and drinks that you normally buy, your shopping bill may even drop slightly). If you decide to include organic produce, this may increase your outlay (although if you are a keen gardener – or know some keen gardeners – you should be able to get some fresh organic produce for little or nothing).

If you choose to buy oils and herbs at health-food or bodycare shops instead of from Neal's Yard Remedies, you will probably have to buy larger amounts than you need, but you would then have oils and herbs you could carry on using for several months.

Overall, depending on what you already have in your food cupboard and bathroom cabinet, the extra cost per day of following *Ten Days To Better Health* should be no more than the cost of a packet of cigarettes or glossy magazine. In comparison with what many people spend on alcohol, tobacco, entertainment, gambling, petrol and sweets each week, this would seem a small price for making a substantial investment in your long-term health.

Getting Started

There is an old proverb which says that getting out of the front door is 90 per cent of the journey, so if you have already decided to try *Ten Days To Better Health* the sooner you start preparing for it the better. In a busy life, waiting for 'the right time' to start something often means putting it off indefinitely, and it is usually far more effective to start where you are rather than wait until you are somewhere you would rather be. After all, it is where you are that gave you the motivation to change your life for the better in the first place.

If you are still undecided whether the programme is for you or not, remember that being healthy in today's world often takes more initial effort than being unhealthy, but it lasts longer. Learning to use your own self-healing power frees you from dependency on others and enables you to be your own life mechanic, caring for your body, mind and spirit and maintaining your health through your own efforts. It can be difficult to decide to make yourself the centre of your own attention for as long as ten days, and you may feel that spending so much time on improving your health is selfish. But if people depend on you, there is no sense in continuing to live in a way that actually makes you less dependable in the long run. Your ability to help others depends on your willingness to devote enough of your time and resources to being healthy yourself.

The short questionnaire on page 35 is designed to help you assess your current situation. It lists twelve different aspects of your life and asks you to give each of them a score between 0 and 100 to show how satisfied you are with each particular aspect. 0 would mean you were totally dissatisfied, 100 would mean you were completely satisfied.

After you have filled it in, mark your answers on the charts on page 36 by drawing vertical lines. For example, if your scores were as follows:

1. Your diet   20
2. Your sleep   50
3. Your level of physical activity   10
4. The amount of time you get to relax   55
5. The amount of time you get to yourself   40
6. The amount of time you spend outdoors   10
7. Your energy level   30
8. Your general health   50
9. Your memory and concentration   60
10. Your work/regular daily activities   40
11. How peaceful you feel   50
12. How happy you are   30

You would mark the Charts like this, using Chart A for questions 1 to 6 and Chart B for Questions 7 to 12:

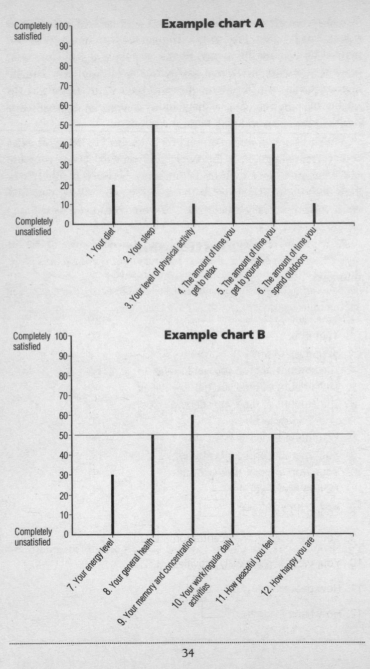

Example chart A

Completely satisfied 100

Completely unsatisfied 0

1. Your diet
2. Your sleep
3. Your level of physical activity
4. The amount of time you get to relax
5. The amount of time you get to yourself
6. The amount of time you spend outdoors

Example chart B

Completely satisfied 100

Completely unsatisfied 0

7. Your energy level
8. Your general health
9. Your memory and concentration
10. Your work/regular daily activities
11. How peaceful you feel
12. How happy you are

Compare the appearance of your Chart A (questions 1 to 6) with your Chart B (questions 7 to 12). Though we tend to attribute poor general health, lack of energy, poor concentration and feelings of tension or anxiety to external circumstances, for most of us there is a direct relationship between our overall sense of wellbeing and the quality of our sleep, diet, activity and relaxation. It is hard to feel healthy when you are tired, tense and poorly nourished.

Charts like these have no absolute meaning, but they provide a simple way of looking at your current situation. Scores on *either* chart less than 50, or one chart showing much lower scores overall than the other, suggest that you would benefit from taking stock and introducing new, healthier patterns into your daily life.

Questionnaire

How satisfied are you with the following aspects of your life? Choose a number between 0 and 100, 0 meaning completely unsatisfied, 100 meaning you are completely satisfied:

1. Your diet ☐

2. Your sleep ☐

3. Your level of physical activity ☐

4. The amount of time you get to relax ☐

5. The amount of time you get to yourself ☐

6. The amount of time you spend outdoors ☐

7. Your energy level ☐

8. Your general health ☐

9. Your memory and concentration ☐

10. Your work/regular daily activities ☐

11. How peaceful you feel ☐

12. How happy you are ☐

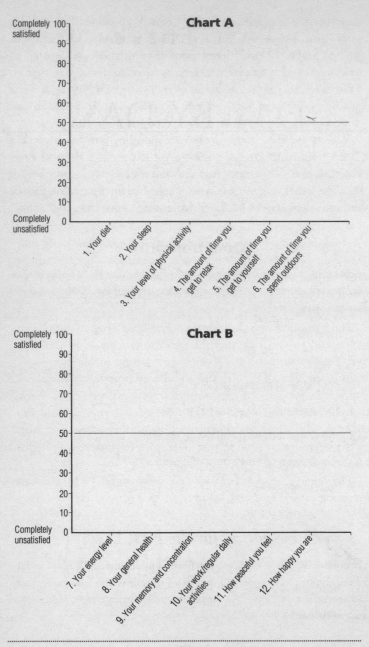

Chart A

Completely satisfied 100

90

80

70

60

50

40

30

20

10

Completely unsatisfied 0

1. Your diet
2. Your sleep
3. Your level of physical activity
4. The amount of time you get to relax
5. The amount of time you get to yourself
6. The amount of time you spend outdoors

Chart B

Completely satisfied 100

90

80

70

60

50

40

30

20

10

Completely unsatisfied 0

7. Your energy level
8. Your general health
9. Your memory and concentration
10. Your work/regular daily activities
11. How peaceful you feel
12. How happy you are

Part Three

DAY BY DAY

꩜

If you have decided to follow the programme, you have hopefully now arranged your quiet space, collected your supplies of herbs and oils, bought in the food you will need according to the lists in Part Two and completed any necessary negotiations with partners, family, friends and work colleagues. If you have, you are ready to start *Ten Days To Better Health*, and we wish you all the best for the next ten days.

This part of the book is made up of ten Daily Programme Guides which lead you step by step through the process of self-healing. Each Guide is laid out in the same way, starting with a brief statement of the aims of the day and a summary timetable. This is followed by a detailed plan containing everything you need to know to follow the programme successfully. Then comes information about the day's herb and essential oil, and finally there is a short 'preparing for tomorrow' section, to help you gather your thoughts for the next day.

The night before you start the programme, read through Preparing for the First Day below.

Preparing for the First Day

Tomorrow you will be using the herb peppermint and the essential oil eucalyptus. Breakfast will consist of muesli with fresh fruit, nuts and seeds, lunch Tabouleh Orientale, and dinner mixed vegetable stew with rice.

Set your alarm for 6.00am and try to get to bed tonight by 10.00pm at the latest. The plan assumes that you do not have to leave for work or start your normal daily activities until 8.00am. If this is not true for you, alter the schedule accordingly so that you wake up two hours before you need to leave for work or start your daily activities. Adjust your bedtime so that you also have at least a full 8 hours in bed.

Your first day will start with a cup of herb tea, followed by a bath or shower (with essential oil), and a short quiet time in your quiet space. You will then make and eat breakfast and – after a short pause to digest – will carry on with Day One – BEGINNINGS.

Wednesday

BEGINNINGS

On the first day, the emphasis is on getting to know a new routine, experiencing new tastes and sensations, and anticipating what is to come.

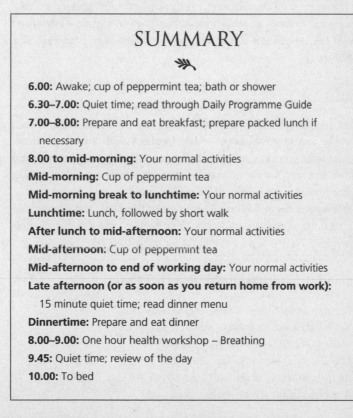

SUMMARY

6.00: Awake; cup of peppermint tea; bath or shower

6.30–7.00: Quiet time; read through Daily Programme Guide

7.00–8.00: Prepare and eat breakfast; prepare packed lunch if necessary

8.00 to mid-morning: Your normal activities

Mid-morning: Cup of peppermint tea

Mid-morning break to lunchtime: Your normal activities

Lunchtime: Lunch, followed by short walk

After lunch to mid-afternoon: Your normal activities

Mid-afternoon: Cup of peppermint tea

Mid-afternoon to end of working day: Your normal activities

Late afternoon (or as soon as you return home from work): 15 minute quiet time; read dinner menu

Dinnertime: Prepare and eat dinner

8.00–9.00: One hour health workshop – Breathing

9.45: Quiet time; review of the day

10.00: To bed

STEP BY STEP

6.00am

Good morning.
Get up slowly and make yourself a cup of peppermint tea: 1 teabag or 1 heaped teaspoon of dried herb to a cup of boiling water; brew for three minutes, strain if necessary. Sit for a few minutes drinking it and waking up gently.

Use the bathroom now, according to your normal routine, but have a warm bath to which you add 5 drops of eucalyptus essential oil diluted in 1 teaspoon of sweet almond oil, just before you step in. If you prefer a shower, put 2 teaspoons of sweet almond oil in a saucer, add 5 drops of eucalyptus oil and rub over your body afterwards. Be careful not to get the oil anywhere near your eyes – it might sting!

6.30am

After you have washed and dressed, go into your quiet space, light a candle and sit down comfortably (perhaps with a blanket round you or over your knees if you feel the cold). Sit quiet and relaxed for ten minutes, letting your mind wander where it will and letting your eyes rest on whatever they find pleasant.

Now read the following Thought for the Day, and then spend five more minutes sitting quietly, reflecting on the words and their meaning.

Thought for the Day

Let all things develop in their natural way
Regard the small as great, regard the few as many
Manage the difficult while they are easy
Manage the great while they are small
All difficult things in the world start from the easy
And great things start from the small

A great tree arises from a tender shoot
A tall building is raised from a heap of earth
A journey of a thousand miles begins from the spot under your feet

LAO TSU

φ

Get up, have a stretch and a yawn, and then look briefly through the rest of this Day Guide, concentrating on the breakfast and lunch menus. When you have collected your thoughts, leave your quiet space and make breakfast.

7.00am–8.00am: Breakfast (plus prepare packed lunch if necessary)

Breakfast Menu 1 glass of unsweetened fruit juice or spring water • muesli with fruits, nuts and seeds

You will need (per person):
1 portion sugar-free muesli base
2 tbs mixed nuts and seeds (e.g. walnut, hazelnut, almond, pine kernels, sunflower, sesame, melon seeds
2 dried dates, chopped
2 dried apricots, chopped
5 tbs chopped mixed fresh fruit/berries, as available
1 portion soya milk

Mix the nuts, dates and apricots with the muesli base, sprinkle the fresh fruit on top and serve with soya milk to taste. Sweeten with a little honey or maple syrup if preferred.

❧ Health Notes

Dried apricots are a good source of selenium, iron and potassium. Dates also contain selenium, iron, zinc and B vitamins. Muesli provides protein, complex carbohydrates, calcium, iron, magnesium, manganese, zinc, B-group vitamins (including biotin and folate) and vitamin E, as

---

well as insoluble fibre. Nuts and seeds are rich in protein, essential polyunsaturated fatty acids, minerals, trace elements, B-vitamins and vitamin E, while fresh fruits and berries add vitamin C, soluble fibre and a variety of vitamins, minerals and trace elements. Soya milk contributes polyunsaturates and amino acids, as well as fibre, vitamins and minerals, and unlike cow's milk it is free of saturated and trans fats. Recent research has confirmed beyond doubt that increasing your daily intake of fresh fruit and unrefined grains protects from cancer, and also from a whole range of 'diseases of civilization', including heart disease, diverticulitis, haemorrhoids and gallstones.

After you have finished your breakfast, sit quietly for five minutes before doing anything else, if possible.

If you need to prepare a packed lunch, refer to the recipe below (page 43). Remember to include some peppermint teabags (or some dried peppermint leaves) for your mid-morning and afternoon breaks, plus a couple of pieces of fruit or some dried fruit if you like to snack. Remember also that it is important to drink some water whenever you feel thirsty. Overall you should be drinking about 1½ litres of water each day (the equivalent of one large bottle of still mineral water per day).

8.00am to mid-morning

Your normal daily activities.

Mid-morning break

A cup of peppermint tea. If you feel hungry, have some fresh or dried fruit.

Mid-morning break to lunchtime

Your normal daily activities.

Lunchtime

Lunch Menu Tabouleh Orientale

You will need (per person):
50 grams/2oz couscous grains (dry weight)
1 tbs safflower oil
¼ red pepper chopped into small cubes
1 tomato, chopped into small cubes
1 spring onion (or ½ small onion), finely chopped
a small handful of lettuce (preferably iceberg), finely chopped
sprig of fresh mint, finely chopped
sprig of fresh parsley, finely chopped
1 tbs lemon juice
salt and pepper to taste

Put 75mls of water and ¼ tsp salt into a small saucepan and bring to the boil. Add the couscous grains and remove from heat. Stir once and set aside while you clean and chop the other ingredients. Stir the safflower oil into the cooled couscous, transfer to a salad bowl, add the other ingredients and mix gently before serving.

⚘ **Health Notes**

Couscous grains are a source of energy and protein, as well as magnesium, iron, zinc, copper, manganese, selenium and B-group vitamins. Safflower oil is an excellent source of essential fatty acids and antioxidant vitamin E. Tomatoes and red peppers are rich in antioxidant vitamin A, and both red and green peppers and tomatoes contain vitamin C and vitamin B6. Spring onions provide calcium, lettuce contains a variety of vitamins and minerals (including vitamins A and E) and both parsley and mint contain calcium and antioxidant vitamins in addition to medicinal substances. Lemons contain vitamin C and calcium, and the dish as a whole is a good source of fibre.

After lunch, sit quietly for five minutes if possible, and then take a short walk outside (preferably in a park or green space if there is one nearby). While you are walking, try and keep your eyes focused into the distance rather than on the path just in front of you, and let your mind wander instead of concentrating on anything in particular. Whatever sort of environment you are in, try and spot at least three things around you that you consider beautiful as you walk.

After lunch to mid-afternoon

Your normal daily activities.

Mid-afternoon break

A cup of peppermint tea (plus a piece of fresh or dried fruit if you feel hungry).

Mid-afternoon to end of the working day

Your normal daily activities.

Late afternoon (or as soon as you return home from work)

Spend fifteen minutes in your quiet space, sitting or lying down quietly. Take a glass of water, unsweetened fruit juice or vegetable juice with you to drink if you feel thirsty. Before you leave your quiet space, read through the recipe below to collect your thoughts for preparing dinner.

Dinnertime

Dinner Menu Mixed vegetable stew with rice

You will need (per person):
150 grams/6oz long grain brown rice (dry weight)
2 tbs olive oil
½ tsp basil
½ tsp ground coriander seeds

½ tsp ground cumin seeds

1 bay leaf

½ tsp tumeric

1 clove garlic, chopped fine or crushed

½ onion, chopped

200 g/7oz of mixed fresh seasonal root vegetables (e.g., carrot, potato, parsnip, celeriac), chopped into medium-sized chunks

50g/2oz dried red lentils, rinsed

1 tomato (skinned or tinned), chopped

1 stick celery, chopped

¼ green pepper, chopped

200mls/8fl oz water or vegetable stock (if using a stock cube, make sure it does not contain monosodium glutamate – 621 – an additive known to cause allergic reactions in some people)

1 tsp lemon juice

salt and pepper to taste

Rinse the rice and put in a medium saucepan with double the volume of cold water. Bring to the boil, then simmer gently (covered) until cooked (approximately 30 to 40 minutes). Stir gently from time to time to make sure the rice does not stick to the bottom of the pan, adding a little extra water if necessary.

While the rice is cooking, heat the oil gently in a large pot or wok. Add the herbs and spices, then the garlic and onion, and stir-fry gently for a few minutes before adding the root vegetables and the lentils. Continue cooking for another minute before adding the peppers, celery and tomato. Add the vegetable stock, then simmer gently (covered), stirring occasionally, until the lentils and root vegetables are tender (20–30 mins). Add the lemon juice, season to taste and serve with a portion of boiled rice. **Keep the left over rice in the fridge for use tomorrow.**

⤳ Health Notes

Wholegrain rice is an excellent source of protein, complex carbohydrate and fibre, as well as magnesium, zinc, copper, manganese and vitamins B1 and B3. Red lentils provide iron, zinc, copper, selenium, vitamin B6 and pantothenic acid. Root vegetables as a group offer antioxidant vitamins A, C and E, plus B vitamins, trace elements, protein, fibre and complex carbohydrate. Celery is a good source of selenium, and calcium is found in onions, lemon juice and the herbs and spices (which also contain a range of vitamins, minerals and trace elements).

Try and sit quietly for a few minutes after your meal before clearing and washing up.

8.00–9.00pm

Health Workshop 1 · BREATHING

This workshop is designed to help you get the most out of the air you breathe.

1 Sit on an upright chair with your hands by your sides, your back straight and both feet on the floor. Close your eyes, then yawn a couple of times. Feel what happens to your mouth, chest and stomach as the yawn develops.

You will notice three things which are fundamental to good breathing. First, since your mouth opens wide, there is plenty of room for air to get in to your lungs. Second, as the yawn starts, your stomach is pushed outwards. Third, as your stomach pushes out, your chest expands. Try yawning once more to make sure.

People tend to think of the lungs as filling the space under the front of the upper chest, but in fact most lung tissue is found in the space at the *back* of the chest. Even though the lungs fill most of the space between the top of the back and the bottom of the rib-cage, many of us use only a small proportion of our lungs to breathe with and only fill up the rest with fresh air when we yawn, or take a very deep breath.

2 Let your hands rest on each side of your chest, fingers in line with the bottom of your rib-cage, thumbs pointing backwards towards your spine. Take a deep breath. You will find your hands being pushed outwards as air fills your lungs all the way down to the bottom. Repeat.

To make full use of your lung capacity, you have to learn to use your diaphragm since it is the diaphragm which is responsible for filling the depths of your lungs. The diaphragm is a large muscle at the bottom of the chest which separates the breathing apparatus from the digestive organs. It moves up and down like a giant plunger as you breathe, sucking air in and then pushing it out as required.

3 Lie down on a bed or mat, a pillow under your head, hands resting lightly on your stomach. Open your mouth a little, close your eyes and take a slow, gentle, deep breath in, then relax and let it out. As you breathe in, the diaphragm moves downwards inside you to suck air in and your stomach gets pushed outwards. As you relax to breathe out, the diaphragm moves upwards into the chest cavity, pushing air up and out and causing your stomach to be pulled in.

Try taking two or three more deep breaths until the feeling becomes clear – breathe in, stomach out; breathe out, stomach in. Now rest for a minute. (If you feel at all light-headed at any point during the rest of this workshop, just stop and breathe normally for a couple of minutes before continuing. Getting a lot of fresh air into your lungs can feel a little unusual at first.)

4 Now you have got your diaphragm moving properly, you can start to exercise it and bring it more under your control. Still lying down comfortably – but now with your arms relaxed by your sides – take three slow deep breaths. Count up to nine in your head as you breathe in, and back down to one again as you breathe out. Leave a count of three between each breath. As you breathe in, push your tummy out slowly and smoothly to encourage the diaphragm to fill your lungs from the bottom up.

As you breathe out, pull your tummy in slowly and progressively to help your diaphragm push as much air out as possible by the end of the breath. Rest for a couple of minutes.

5 Practise emptying your lungs completely by going '*huh*' four or five times without taking a breath in between. See how much air you can actually squeeze out of your chest. Rest for a minute.

Now repeat Exercise 4, counting like before and filling and emptying your lungs as completely as possible. Try and feel your lungs filling up from bottom to top, then emptying from top to bottom. On the in breath, only your stomach should be moving on counts 1 to 6. The top part of your chest should be still to start with and only expand on counts 7, 8 and 9. As you breathe out, let your upper chest fall first *before* you start pulling your stomach in to push out the air. The whole sequence should be as smooth as possible, without any jerkiness or hesitation. The change between the in breath and the out breath should also be smooth, with no pause.

Rest for a minute.

Sit up slowly, wait for a few seconds then stand up and stretch a bit before doing the last exercise in this workshop.

6 Stand relaxed, feet planted firmly on the floor a little apart, arms hanging loosely by your sides. Take a breath in to a count of nine (using your diaphragm as before), then open your mouth WIDE and sing a low pitched '*aaah*' sound as you count back down to one. Rest.

It doesn't matter what the *ahhh* sounds like. What counts is that it is low, relaxed and as even as possible. The aim is to make a sound which doesn't falter or change in volume as you start to run out of air.

Try this again two or three times, making sure that your shoulders don't lift up towards your neck as you breathe in. If you're using your diaphragm properly, the only movement you should feel as you breathe in deeply is your stomach pushing down and out and the front of your chest rising slightly. Remember to open your mouth wide, and to keep it open until you have counted all the way back to one.

That's the end of the practical part of this first workshop. In it, you have explored the full capacity of your lungs, felt your diaphragm moving, and realized that a full deep breath involves using your diaphragm to fill your lungs from the bottom up. Efficient breathing does not involve big movements of the chest, and never requires lifting of the shoulders.

You will probably have found that the hardest part was keeping each breath smooth and even, but with just a little regular practice you will gain more control over your diaphragm and be able to breathe more fully, calmly and efficiently without even thinking about it.

From now on, you will do a couple of breathing exercises each morning before your bath or shower, but you can practise anywhere, anytime if you want. The only thing to remember is not to overdo it. Make sure you have a proper rest in between each exercise sequence, and keep your practice sessions short.

Before leaving this health workshop, read through the notes below about today's herb and oil, and then look through the 'Preparing for Tomorrow' section.

Today's Herb · PEPPERMINT *(Mentha piperita)*

Mint has been used as a medicine for thousands of years and has a history that can be traced back to Egyptian times. It is cooling and soothing and reduces mental and emotional tension by relaxing the body and clearing the mind. It is thus an excellent substitute for tea and coffee, and a good herb to use during times of change. In traditional herbalism it represents light, perception, intelligence and harmony and promotes truth, humility and good in all. As a medicine, it relieves most digestive ailments and is useful for calming nausea and morning, travel and sea sickness. It can also be helpful in migraine and to ease breathing in chest complaints. A pot of peppermint tea added to a bath can reduce itching from eczema.

Today's Oil · EUCALYPTUS *(Eucalyptus globulus)*

Native Australians used eucalyptus as a disinfectant and to cool fevers. Immigrants quickly learned to use it too, and it is now popular all over the world. The essential oil has a refreshing, calming and cooling effect and relieves exhaustion, confusion and anxiety. Useful in times of change, it increases concentration and mental clarity. It is an excellent antiseptic and natural antibiotic which can be used in massage oil, inhalations and baths to cleanse, stimulate and revitalise the body and the mind. A few drops of eucalyptus in a little warm water makes a good antiseptic gargle and mouthwash, and for skin infections, wounds, ulcers and insect bites a little oil can be applied directly (though sparingly – it is a strong oil and may sting) to the affected area. A few drops of oil in sweet almond oil can be rubbed over sore joints to ease stiffness and discomfort, and 10–15 drops in a sitz bath (see Appendix) can be used to help treat genito-urinary infections. To clear the airways and ease breathing in sinus and chest complaints, put 10–15 drops of eucalyptus oil in a bowl, add some boiling water, place a towel over your head and inhale the steam for 5–10 minutes.

φ

PREPARING FOR TOMORROW

Tomorrow you will be using the herb fennel and the essential oil marjoram. Breakfast will be muesli with fruits, nuts and seeds, lunch a rice salad with French dressing and dinner a baked potato and fennel dish. Set your alarm tonight for 6.00am (or two hours before you leave for work/start your normal daily activities). Day Two – CHANGING will start with a cup of fennel tea, some breathing exercises, a bath or shower with essential oil and morning quiet time.

9.45–10.00pm

Before going to bed, go once more into your quiet space and sit quietly. Breathe deeply in and out a couple of times, then look back over the day in your mind's eye. Consider the things you did that you feel good about, and remember also anything that happened – or that was said – which you don't feel so good about. See what you can learn from the day's experiences, then let them go. Life is a mixture of what we call good and bad, but happiness comes from not being thrown off-balance by either. Reviewing the events of the day – giving yourself credit for the good you have done and forgiveness for any bad done or done to you – is an important part of learning to live in the present. Yesterday is buried in today. Tomorrow is created by your current action.

Sleep well.

CHANGING

On the second day, there is a growing awareness of the impact of past stresses on bodily health and function.

SUMMARY

6.00: Awake; breathing exercise; cup of fennel tea; bath or shower

6.30–7.00: Quiet time; read through Daily Programme Guide

7.00–8.00: Prepare and eat breakfast; prepare packed lunch if necessary

Mid-morning: Cup of fennel tea

Lunchtime: Lunch, followed by short walk

Mid-afternoon: Cup of fennel tea

Late afternoon (or as soon as you return home from work): 15 minute quiet time; read dinner menu

Dinnertime: Prepare and eat dinner

8.00–9.00: One hour health workshop – Stretching

9.45: Quiet time; review of the day

10.00: To bed

STEP BY STEP

6.00am

Before you get out of bed, take three long, slow, deep breaths in and out (remembering to use your diaphragm) and then lie still for a minute, breathing quietly. Get up slowly, and make yourself a cup of fennel tea – 1 teabag or 1 teaspoon of dried seeds to a cup of boiling water – brew for a few minutes, strain if necessary.

After your tea, use the bathroom and have a warm bath or shower, using the sweet marjoram oil in the same way as yesterday's eucalyptus oil.

6.30am

When you have washed and dressed, go into your quiet space, light a candle and sit quiet and relaxed for 10 minutes. As you are sitting, let your attention rest for a few seconds on different parts of your body, sensing whether they are warm or cold, tense or relaxed. Try the following sequence: Centre of the chest ▶ right foot ▶ left hand ▶ top of head ▶ bottom of the spine ▶ centre of forehead ▶ navel ▶ back of neck ▶ right hand ▶ left foot ▶ centre of chest.

Now read the following Thought for the Day, and then spend five more minutes sitting quietly.

Thought for the Day

The essence of success in any project is to know exactly what you want, and then to direct all your actions towards achieving it. Anything you do which does not in some way help you towards your goal makes it more difficult to reach.

THE PHI BOOK

φ

Get up and have a stretch. Then take a slow deep breath in and, on the out breath, sing a gentle, low pitched *ahhh* sound (as you did in the workshop last night). Sit down again and have a look through the rest of this Daily Programme Guide, concentrating on the breakfast and lunch menus. When you have collected your thoughts, leave your quiet space and make breakfast.

7.00–8.00am: Breakfast (plus prepare packed lunch if necessary)

Breakfast Menu A glass of unsweetened fruit juice or spring water • muesli with fruits, nuts and seeds

You will need (per person):
1 portion sugar-free muesli base
2 tbs mixed nuts and seeds
2 dried dates, chopped
2 dried apricots, chopped
5 tbs chopped mixed fresh fruit/berries, as available
1 portion soya milk

Mix the nuts, dates and apricots with the muesli base, sprinkle the fresh fruit on top and serve with soya milk to taste. Sweeten with a little maple syrup or honey if preferred.

⚛ **Health Notes**

Naturopathic nutrition involves increasing your daily intake of plant based foods, because plants contain all the nutrients necessary for human health and vitality in a natural, tasty, low cost, easy-to-prepare form. They are high in fibre, low in cholesterol, contain no saturated or trans fats and are rich in health giving polyunsaturated fatty acids and antioxidant vitamins and minerals. They contain no refined sugar, provide all the essential amino acids and essential fatty acids we need, and are our only dietary source of energy-giving complex carbohydrates.

After you have finished your breakfast, sit quietly for a few minutes before doing anything else.

If you need to prepare a packed lunch, refer to the recipes below. Remember to take some fennel tea (plus some fruit or dried fruit) for your morning and afternoon breaks, as well as bottled water if necessary.

Mid-morning break

A cup of fennel tea. If you feel hungry, have some fresh or dried fruit.

Lunchtime

Lunch Menu Rice salad with French dressing

You will need (per person):
cooked brown rice (left over from yesterday's dinner)
½ spring onion, sliced
1 stalk celery, sliced
¼ red pepper, chopped in small cubes
1 small carrot, grated
2 dried apricots, chopped finely
¼ fennel, chopped finely
1 tbs mixed nuts and seeds (e.g., walnut, brazil, sunflower, sesame)

Put all the salad ingredients in a bowl and mix well. **Set aside a portion (about one third) of the mixed salad and keep in the fridge for use in this evening's meal.**

For the dressing (enough to last several days):
5 tbs safflower oil
5 tbs walnut oil
juice of ½ lemon
1 clove of garlic, peeled and left whole with a cross cut in one end
1 tbs tahini (optional)
1 tbs maple syrup
1 tbs soya sauce
1 tsp French mustard
salt and pepper to taste

Put all the dressing ingredients into a jam jar, put the lid on and shake well.

Mix some dressing in with the rice salad to taste and serve. (If you prefer a more spicy dressing, add some cumin, coriander, bay leaf and a pinch of cayenne. You could also add some dried mixed herbs.)

₩ Health Notes

A total raw food diet is not a practical proposition for many people these days, but there are a number of benefits to be gained from eating some foods raw each day. Heating destroys the living cells that make up fresh plant foods, and this reduces their vitality and depletes them of some important nutrients. Vitamin C, thiamin and folic acid are destroyed by heating, and high temperatures will also denature vitamin A and vitamin E (both important antioxidants). From the naturopathic point of view, the fact that all food provided directly by nature is raw – and that every other species on the planet survives very well on it – is a good reason to eat at least one raw food meal a day. Raw food diets can also be helpful in the management of a variety of illnesses including diabetes, arthritis and cancer.

After lunch, sit quietly for five minutes before taking your midday walk. Remember to relax your eyes by keeping them focused into the distance as you walk, and to notice things around you that you find beautiful or pleasing in some way.

Mid-afternoon break

A cup of fennel tea (plus a piece of fresh or dried fruit if you feel hungry).

Late afternoon (or as soon as you return home from work)

Spend fifteen minutes in your quiet space, sitting or lying down quietly. Take a glass of water, unsweetened fruit juice or vegetable juice with you to drink if you feel thirsty. Before leaving your quiet space, read through the dinner recipe below.

Dinnertime

Dinner Menu Baked potato and fennel dish with stir-fried rice

You will need (per person):
500g/1lb 2oz potatoes, cut in quarters
1 tsp olive oil
½ fennel, sliced
½ red onion, sliced
1–2 tomatoes, sliced
½ lemon, sliced thinly
1 small handful of parsley, chopped
60mls vegetable stock
salt and pepper to taste

Parboil the potatoes in lightly salted water until they are just tender, meanwhile preparing the other ingredients. Grease an ovenproof dish with the olive oil, arrange *half* the potatoes on the bottom (**setting the rest aside to keep in the fridge for use tomorrow**) then add the other vegetables in layers – fennel, onion, tomatoes and finally lemon on top. Sprinkle with chopped parsley and some salt and pepper, add the water or stock, cover with foil and bake for 30–40 minutes at 200°C/400°F/gas mark 6. Then, 5 minutes before serving, take the rice salad left over from lunch and stir-fry it in a little olive oil as an accompaniment.

﹋ **Health Notes**

Potatoes are a marvellous source of energy, protein and fibre, as well as vitamins and minerals including vitamin C, vitamins B1, B3 and B6, folate, pantothenic acid and potassium. Fennel has a soothing, calming effect on the digestion and improves the digestion of fatty foods. It also contains potassium, zinc, vitamin B3 and folic acid. Parsley is rich in vitamins A and C, and in iron, calcium, magnesium and manganese. Vitamin C helps us to absorb iron from the digestive tract into the bloodstream.

Sit quietly for a few minutes after your meal before clearing and washing up.

8.00–9.00pm

Health Workshop 2 · STRETCHING

Stress causes muscle tension, and muscle tension can cause a variety of unpleasant symptoms such as headaches, backache and muscle cramps. Tense muscles interfere with the free flow of blood around the body and, since contracting muscles use up energy, muscle tension can also be an important cause of general tiredness and low vitality. Stretching muscles helps them to relax, and also helps relieve the emotional or mental difficulties that caused them to become tense in the first place.

The following exercises are designed to help you stretch all the main muscle groups in your body, paying special attention to the neck and shoulders. They will help you to let go of muscle tensions and the difficulties they represent, and will leave you feeling relaxed and energized. Before you begin, lay out your blanket or mat on the floor to do the exercises on, take off your shoes and make sure that the clothes you are wearing are comfortable and loose fitting, to allow you to bend and stretch easily.

Read each exercise through a couple of times before doing it, rehearsing the movements in your mind's eye. Then try the exercise *slowly* and carefully, allowing your muscles time to stretch but without causing strain or discomfort. Read through the exercise again to check the movements, then repeat the exercise without looking at the text. Groan freely as you stretch and don't forget to breathe! Fitness and flexibility vary greatly from one person to another, so if your joint mobility is restricted for any reason, and you feel that some of the movements may be too taxing, don't worry. Simply do what you can do comfortably and make sure you only stretch to your own comfortable limit, and not beyond. With stretching, every little helps.

Exercise I

Stand relaxed, feet slightly apart. Put your hands together palm to palm in front of you, fingers interlocked, then stretch your arms up over your head. Still holding your hands together over your head, stretch the muscles on the right side of your body by bending slowly sideways to the left. Then stretch your left side by bending sideways to the right. Stretch twice more to each side, then let your arms hang down by your sides and relax.

Exercise II

1 Still standing relaxed, feet slightly apart, put your hands together palm to palm – fingers interlocked – and put your arms out in front of you. Keeping your shoulders down, stretch your arms as far forward as you can to loosen up the muscles between your shoulder blades.

2 Now lower your head between your outstretched arms, curling your neck and upper back forwards slightly. Move your folded hands to the back of your neck, and then draw your elbows up and back as far as you can.

3 Let your hands go, then give a deep sigh as you straighten up and let your arms hang down by your sides. Relax for a minute.

Exercise III

1 Hold your hands behind your back, fingers interlocked, and stretch your arms downwards and away from your back while you lift your chest forward and up, arching your spine and looking upwards and backwards as far as you can.

2 Let your hands go, straighten your back and neck, look ahead and stand relaxed for a minute.

Exercise IV

1 Stand with your arms by your sides, feet a little apart, and take a deep, slow breath in and out.

2 Lower your head very slowly forwards until your chin touches your chest.

3 Continue to bend forwards (remembering to breathe), curving your back slowly and progressively from the top downwards and keeping your lower back straight for as long as possible. Your head and arms should hang down loose and heavy as you continue to bend.

4 When your fingertips are at the same level as your knees, bend your knees a little so that you can continue bending progressively forward until you can touch the floor (or as near as possible).

5 Relax your facial muscles and take two deep breaths in and out.

6 Unfold yourself by uncurling your back from the bottom upwards, breathing deeply and sighing as you breathe out. Feel your vertebrae 'stacking' one on top of the other as you straighten up.

7 Stand upright, hands hanging loosely by your sides and relax for a minute.

Exercise V

1a Stand with your back to a wall, about a foot away from it.

2a Take a deep breath in and, as you breathe out, turn your left foot outwards slightly and hold your arms up in front of you (as if you were in a 'hold-up'), hands at same level as your shoulders, palms facing forwards.

3a Breathe in again and as you breathe out, start turning your upper body to the left and continue to turn (letting your knees bend as necessary) until you are facing the wall behind you. Keep your head in line with your shoulders as you turn.

4a Put your palms on the wall, then turn your head even further round, looking as far over your left shoulder as you can without strain.

5a Remember to breathe while you stay in this position for a few seconds.

6a Take a deep breath in, and as you breathe out start untwisting yourself again – first your head, then your shoulders, then your middle-back, then your lower back until you get back to the position you started in (and with your left foot parallel to your right again).

1b Repeat the exercise twisting to the right, i.e.:

2b Take a deep breath in and as you breathe out, turn your right foot outwards slightly and hold your arms up in front of you, hands at the same level as your shoulders, palms facing forwards.

3b Breathe in again and, as you breathe out, start turning your upper body to the right and continue to turn (letting your knees bend as necessary) until you are facing the wall behind you. Keep your head in line with your shoulders as you turn.

4b Put your palms on the wall, then turn your head even further round, looking as far over your right shoulder as you can without strain.

5b Remember to breathe while you stay in this position for a few seconds.

6b Take a deep breath in, and as you breathe out start untwisting yourself again – first your head, then your shoulders, then your middle back, then your lower back until you get back to the position you started in (and with your right foot parallel to your left again). Return your hands to your sides, and relax for a minute.

Exercise VI

1 Sit on an upright chair (e.g. a dining chair).

2 Grip under the sides of the seat with both hands, in line with your hips.

3 Straighten your back and push your chest forward.

4 Let go of the chair with your left hand, and curl your left arm over the top of your head so that your left hand covers your right ear.

5 Then lean your head to the left and, still holding on under the seat with your right hand, *gently* pull your head down towards your left shoulder. Remember to breathe.

6 Straighten up, then repeat the exercise the other way round (i.e. with your left hand holding under the seat and your right hand placed over your left ear, easing your head down towards your right shoulder). Relax for a minute.

Exercise VII

1 Stand upright with your feet a little apart, arms hanging down loosely by your sides.

2 Move your hands up in front of your heart, elbows bent, and palms together.

3 As you take a slow deep breath in, lift your arms upwards as far as you can reach, palms still together.

4 As you breathe out, move your hands apart, outwards and backwards in a big circle, ending up with your palms meeting in front of your heart again.

5 Stand still for a little while, breathe gently and relax.

6 Repeat the exercise once more.

Exercise VIII

1 Stand upright and take a deep breath in.

2 As you breathe out, bend forwards from the hips as far as you can without bending your knees, keeping your back straight and letting your arms hang down loosely in front of you.

3 Stay in this position a little while, breathing quietly and feeling the stretch at the back of your legs.

4 Straighten up slowly and relax for a minute.

Exercise IX (optional)

1 Stand upright and take a deep breath in. As you breathe out, bend forwards from the hips as far as you can, this time bending your knees so that you can touch the floor in front of your feet with your hands.

2 With your fingers on the floor to keep you balanced, take a big step backwards with your right leg, stretching it out as far behind you as possible, underside of the toes touching the ground.

3 Now push your chest forwards, lift your head, and look up and back as far as you can. Remember to breathe.

4 Come out of the position slowly by lowering your head, bringing your right leg forwards, placing your right foot beside the left and standing up slowly. Relax a moment.

5 Repeat the exercise, but this time take the backwards step with your *left* leg. When you have finished, relax for a minute.

Exercise X

1 Sit down on the floor with your legs straight out in front of you.

2 Take a deep breath and, as you breathe out, lean forwards slowly keeping your back and your legs straight and letting your hands glide down the tops of your legs until you can't bend forward any further.

3 Stay in this position for a moment, breathing quietly, then slowly sit up straight again.

Exercise XI

1 Still sitting down on the floor, bend your knees to the sides and bring the soles of your feet together in front of you, as close to your bottom as possible.

2 Hold on to your feet with your hands, then very gently jiggle your knees up and down for a few moments, keeping your back straight.

3 Straighten your legs out in front of you and relax for a minute.

Exercise XII

1 Lie flat on your back (with a blanket over you if you wish), arms by your sides, feet a little apart. If you have a bad back, you may find it more comfortable to bend your knees, resting the soles of your feet just in front of your bottom.

2 Try to relax your whole body, one part at a time, starting at the feet and working upwards.

3 When you have rested comfortably for a few minutes, sit up slowly.

Before leaving this health workshop, read through the notes below about today's herb and oil, and then look through the 'Preparing For Tomorrow' section.

Today's Herb · FENNEL *(Foeniculum vulgare)*

Fennel has been used as a culinary and medicinal herb since ancient times and has the reputation of bringing strength, courage and long life to those who use it. Its calming and soothing properties encourage relaxation, communication and self-expression, and fennel is also an excellent remedy for indigestion, bloating and wind. It increases milk production in nursing mothers and, since its soothing properties are passed on in the milk, it can benefit both mother and baby by easing stress and calming colic. It can also be used for catarrhal conditions and as a gentle expectorant to ease coughs. A compress made with fresh fennel tea can also be used to cheer up tired or sore eyes.

Today's Oil · SWEET MARJORAM
(*Origanum marjorana*)

Marjoram is a warming, comforting and relaxing herb and a valuable aid to overcoming the effects of stress and overwork. Like fennel, it encourages communication and creative expression, and can be used for all problems related to tension or coldness such as period pain, indigestion, high blood pressure, tension headache, sore muscles and arthritis. Its relaxing effects on the mind and body can also help to relieve anxiety and ease insomnia. It is a useful first-aid remedy, providing relief for sprains and bruises and easing rheumatic aches and pains. For massage, use 5 drops of marjoram oil in 10mls (2 tsp) of sweet almond oil.

φ

PREPARING FOR TOMORROW

Tomorrow you will be using the herb thyme and the essential oil pine. Breakfast will be a fruit salad of mixed fresh and dried fruits, lunch a potato salad with tahini dressing, and dinner baked vegetables with a mushroom sauce. Set your alarm tonight as usual – 6.00am or two hours before you leave for work or start your normal daily activities. Day Three – CLEANSING will start with a cup of thyme tea, some stretching exercises, a bath or shower with essential oil, and morning quiet time.

9.45–10.00pm

Before going to bed, go into your quiet space and sit quietly. Breathe deeply in and out a couple of times, and then turn over the events of the day in your mind. Be pleased for what went well, gain strength from what went badly, and then try to let go of both. Hanging on to the past takes energy and releasing it frees this energy for us to use to be healthier and happier. If you find it hard to let go of the day's events, try imagining that your heart is a bright, beautiful fire into which you put your daily experiences one by one, consuming and transforming each of them into light.

Tomorrow morning you are going to start a 'Dream Diary'. Take a notebook and pen to bed with you tonight and, the moment you wake up, write down any dreams (or parts of dreams) that you can remember.

Sleep well.

CLEANSING

On the third day, the body, mind and emotions start to release accumulated toxins, thoughts, frustrations and anxieties.

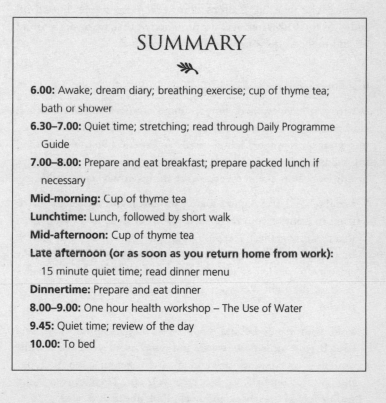

SUMMARY

6.00: Awake; dream diary; breathing exercise; cup of thyme tea; bath or shower

6.30–7.00: Quiet time; stretching; read through Daily Programme Guide

7.00–8.00: Prepare and eat breakfast; prepare packed lunch if necessary

Mid-morning: Cup of thyme tea

Lunchtime: Lunch, followed by short walk

Mid-afternoon: Cup of thyme tea

Late afternoon (or as soon as you return home from work): 15 minute quiet time; read dinner menu

Dinnertime: Prepare and eat dinner

8.00–9.00: One hour health workshop – The Use of Water

9.45: Quiet time; review of the day

10.00: To bed

STEP BY STEP

6.00am

The moment you wake up, write down everything you can remember about the dreams you had last night. Then, before you get out of bed, take three long, slow, deep breaths in and out, and lie still for a moment, breathing quietly. Get up slowly and make yourself a cup of thyme tea – 1 teaspoon of dried leaves or a few fresh sprigs to a cup of boiling water; brew for a few minutes, strain if necessary.

After your tea, use the bathroom and have a warm bath or shower. Use pine oil, 2 drops diluted in 1 tsp sweet almond oil added to the bathwater or 2 drops mixed with 2 tsp sweet almond oil and rubbed into your skin after your shower.

6.30am

When you have washed, put on some comfortable, loose-fitting clothes, take your dream diary and coloured pens or pencils and go into your quiet space. Light a candle and spend five minutes doing the following stretching exercises, which are taken from last night's health workshop. Remember to take things slowly and gently.

1 Stand relaxed, feet slightly apart. Put your hands together palm to palm in front of you, then stretch your arms up over your head (hands still together). Keeping your arms over your head, stretch the muscles on the right side of your body by bending slowly sideways to the left. Then stretch your left side by bending sideways to the right. Let your arms hang down by your sides and relax.

2 Fold your hands behind your back, fingers interlocked, and stretch your arms downwards and away from your back while you lift your chest forwards and up, arching your spine and looking upwards and backwards as far as you can. Then let your hands go, straighten your back and neck, look ahead and relax.

3 Stand with your arms by your sides, feet a little apart. Lower your head very slowly forward until your chin touches your chest, then continue to bend forwards, curving your back slowly and progressively from the top downwards (keeping your lower back straight as long as possible). Your head and arms should hang down loose and heavy as you bend. When your fingertips are at the same level as your knees, unfold yourself by uncurling your back from the bottom upwards, breathing deeply and sighing as you breathe out. Stand upright and relax.

4 Hold your hands up in front of your heart, palms together. As you take a slow deep breath in, lift your arms upwards as far as you can reach, palms still together. As you breathe out, move your hands apart, outwards and backwards in a big circle, ending up with your palms meeting in front of your heart again. Stand still for a moment, breathing gently, then sit down and read the following Thought for the Day before sitting quietly for five minutes.

Thought for the Day

To pour anything into a full bottle, one must first empty out what it contains.

LEO TOLSTOY

φ

Take your dream diary and look through what you wrote when you woke this morning. Don't worry if you didn't write very much – you will find you are able to remember more and more as the week goes on. Broadly speaking, dreams consist of five different types of images: remnants of experiences from the previous day; things that are 'on your mind'; messages from your subconscious to your conscious mind; recurring themes; and the apparently unexplainable. As you read through your notes, mark the different parts of your dreams with a coloured pencil according to the following scheme:

- Red for remnants
- Yellow for things on your mind
- Green for messages
- Blue for recurring themes
- Purple for the apparently unexplainable

Don't spend too long on this – just follow your instinct about which things mean what.

Finally, have a look through the rest of this Daily Programme Guide, concentrating on the breakfast and lunch menus. When you have collected your thoughts, leave your quiet space and make breakfast.

7.00–8.00am: Breakfast (plus prepare lunch if necessary)

Breakfast Menu   1 glass unsweetened fruit juice or spring water • fruit salad with fresh and dried fruits

You will need (per person):
1 small portion seasonal fruits or berries
1 banana, sliced
handful of grapes, halved
½ apple, cored and chopped
3 or 4 dates, stoned and chopped
3 or 4 dried apricots, chopped
5 tbs unsweetened fruit juice

Mix together all the ingredients in a bowl and serve.

⋙   Health Notes

Digesting, absorbing and metabolizing the food we eat uses a considerable amount of energy, and restricting your food intake slightly during a period of healing allows some of this energy to be channelled into the process of healing. Gently cutting down on the food you take in for a couple of days also helps the body to dispose of stored up

---

toxins, and allows the organs responsible for getting rid of waste products (kidneys, liver, skin and lungs) to work more efficiently. From today until Sunday, therefore, you will notice the menus becoming simpler and simpler as a way of encouraging your natural self-cleaning ability.

After you have finished your breakfast, sit quietly for a few minutes before doing anything else.

If you need to prepare a packed lunch, refer to the recipe below. Remember to take some thyme tea (plus some fresh and/or dried fruit) for your morning and afternoon breaks, as well as bottled water if necessary. It is particularly important that you drink plenty of fresh water over the next few days – little and often – to help your body make the most of this period of cleansing.

Mid-morning break

A cup of thyme tea. If you feel hungry, have some fresh or dried fruit.

Lunchtime

Lunch Menu Potato salad with tahini dressing

You will need (per person):
Left over cold boiled potatoes (from yesterday)
½ spring onion (or a small bunch of chives), sliced
1 spear broccoli, divided into small bouquets
¼ red pepper, finely chopped
2 or 3 radishes, sliced
1 tbs tahini mixed with 2 tbs French dressing
Salt and pepper to taste

Put the potatoes and the spring onion in a salad bowl. Add the tahini and French dressing and mix well. Add the broccoli (raw or lightly steamed and cooled, according to taste), then the pepper and radishes and mix again. Serve.

🌿 Health Notes

People making the change to a healthier, more natural way of eating are sometimes concerned that they may not get enough protein in their diet if they increase their intake of plant-based foods. In fact, plants are the fundamental high quality protein source on the planet and contain all the amino acids necessary for health. Modern research has shown that human beings need just 10 per cent or less of their calorie intake to be in the form of protein (human breast milk only contains between 5 and 8 per cent), and nearly all plants contain 10 per cent of their calories as protein. As long as the food you eat is meeting your daily calorie needs, therefore, a plant-based diet will easily meet your protein needs. There is no truth in the suggestion that you have to combine different plant protein sources in a meal to make them 'complete', and plant protein comes naturally packaged with other important nutrients – complex carbohyrates, fibre, vitamins, minerals, trace elements and essential fatty acids. Unlike animal protein sources, plants are naturally low in cholesterol and saturated fats.

After lunch, sit quietly for five minutes before taking your midday walk. If possible, walk somewhere where there is some running water, and spend a quiet minute or two resting your eyes on it before completing your walk.

Mid-afternoon break

A cup of thyme tea (plus a piece of fresh or dried fruit if you feel hungry).

Late afternoon (or as soon as you return home from work):

Spend fifteen minutes in your quiet space, sitting or lying down quietly. Take a glass of water, unsweetened fruit juice or vegetable juice with you if you feel thirsty. Before leaving your quiet space, read through the dinner recipe below:

Dinnertime

Dinner Menu Baked vegetables with mushroom and thyme sauce

> *You will need (per person):*
> 500g/1lb 2oz assorted vegetables (according to season and taste) e.g. potato, sweet potato, parsnip, beetroot, onion, courgette, carrot
> 1 clove garlic
> 2 tbs olive oil
> ½ tsp mixed herbs
> ¼ tsp paprika
> ¼ tsp ground cumin
> ¼ tsp ground coriander
> salt and pepper to taste
>
> **For the sauce:**
> 50g/2oz mushrooms, sliced
> 1 tbs olive oil
> 1 tbs flour
> 8 tbs vegetable stock
> ½ tsp thyme
> 8 tbs soya milk
> salt and pepper to taste

Pre-heat the oven to 180°C/350°F/gas mark 4. Chop the vegetables into big chunks of more or less the same size, and put them in a greased ovenproof dish. Add the whole garlic clove, dab the vegetables with olive oil and sprinkle with the herbs, spices, salt and pepper. Bake for about forty minutes (or until the vegetables are cooked through). As the vegetables are cooking, sauté the mushrooms in olive oil until they give off their liquid, then sprinkle in the flour, stirring continuously, and slowly add the vegetable stock. Bring to the boil then add the thyme and simmer for five minutes. Just before serving, stir in the soya milk and adjust the seasoning. Serve with the baked vegetables.

> ### ↝ Health Notes
>
> As you know, root vegetables as a group contain antioxidant vitamins
> and trace elements as well as protein, fibre and energy-giving complex
> carbohydrates. Beetroot is also an important medicinal plant of partic-
> ular use in chronic conditions involving the blood and immune system.
> Herbs and spices are packed with nutrients – cumin, for example, con-
> tains calcium, magnesium, iron, copper, zinc, vitamin A, vitamins B1,
> B2 and B3 – and have a variety of medicinal properties. Garlic, the
> jewel in the crown of natural medicine, is one of the most effective
> antibiotic and immune-stimulant plants available. Eating garlic regu-
> larly can lower blood pressure, reduce blood cholesterol and decrease
> the tendency of the blood to clot, which makes it useful in the preven-
> tion and management of heart disease.

Sit quietly for a few minutes after your meal before clearing and
washing up.

8.00–9.00pm

Health Workshop 3 · THE USE OF WATER

'There is no such thing as a cure-all; but, if there were, it would be
cold water, properly applied.' So said the eminent naturopath
Dr Henry Lindlahr at the beginning of the century, and the
therapeutic use of water – hydrotherapy – is still one of the most
effective ways of increasing vitality and encouraging healing. This
workshop is designed to stimulate your circulation and improve the
elimination of waste materials from your body, leaving you with a
feeling of warm, gentle invigoration. It consists of two parts: applying the technique, and rest.

You will need:
- A warm bathroom
- A towel or bath mat to stand on

- A sink or bowl full of cold water
- A towel to dry yourself
- A cosy dressing-gown or tracksuit to relax in afterwards

Method:

1 Fill the sink or bowl with cold water.

2 Remove your clothes, and stand on a towel.

3 Dip your hands in the water and rub it over your body, starting with the face and working downwards bit by bit to your feet.

4 Dry yourself with a towel, then repeat the exercise, again starting with the face and working down.

5 Dry yourself again, put on your dressing-gown or tracksuit and then go and lie down comfortably with a blanket over you for half an hour.

This 'hand rub' stimulates circulation through the whole body. The increased blood flow brings improved nutrition to your body cells and helps with the removal of accumulated waste products. The first touch of cold water on your skin may be a slight shock, but a comforting warm feeling soon develops bringing relaxation to mind and body.

Before finishing this health workshop, read through the notes below about today's herb and oil, and then look through the 'Preparing for Tomorrow' section.

Today's Herb · THYME *(Thymus vulgaris)*

Thyme is a warming, sweet, pleasantly aromatic herb blessed with a multitude of therapeutic properties. It is associated with cleansing, courage, grace and energy and its use dates back to ancient Egypt. It is a powerful antiseptic with marked antibiotic properties and can be used internally and externally to treat colds, flu and a variety of bacterial, viral and fungal infections. For chest infections it can be used in steam inhalations (see Appendix, page 177). To ease skin infections, try adding a pot of thyme tea to the bath water. For genito-urinary complaints, a thyme sitz-bath (see Appendix, page 178) can be used in addition to thyme tea. Thyme is also an extremely effective digestive remedy for cramps and diarrhoea.

Today's Oil · PINE *(Pinus sylvestris)*

Pine oil is made from pine resin and is cleansing, refreshing, warming and invigorating. It is stimulating to the nervous system and is helpful where concentration is poor and where old guilt or misunderstandings are making it hard to get free of the past and move on. Like thyme, it is a powerful antiseptic useful in both respiratory and urinary infections (in inhalations and sitz baths), and can be used in foot baths to treat sweaty feet. In massage and bath oils it can be used to ease arthritic pains and muscle tension. Note that pine is a powerful essential oil which should be used sparingly, and always dissolved in another oil (such as sweet almond oil).

φ

PREPARING FOR TOMORROW

Tomorrow you will be using the herb St John's wort and the oil calendula. Breakfast will be a fresh fruit salad, lunch an avocado and grapefruit salad with carrots and mixed greens, and dinner a celeriac and beetroot salad with herbs and fruits. Set your alarm tonight as usual – 6.00am or two hours before you start your normal daily activities – and don't forget your dream diary and a pen. Day Four – HEALING will start with your dream diary, a cup of St John's wort tea, some simple hydrotherapy and morning quiet time.

9.45–10.00pm
Before going to bed, go into your quiet space and sit comfortably. Breathe deeply in and out a couple of times and then review the

day's events as usual. When you have finished, half close your eyes and imagine yourself sitting relaxed beside a clear, bright mountain stream. See the light dancing on the water, hear the rush and gurgle as it passes between the rocks, and sense the calm and peace that always accompany true beauty. Remember that all life emerged from water and that water is the foundation of the body. To quote the great naturalist and scientist Viktor Schauberger, 'Water is the raw material of every culture, and the basis of every bodily and spiritual development.'

Remember to leave your dream diary ready by the bed, and sleep well.

Saturday

HEALING

On the fourth day, you will feel the depth of your accumulated tiredness, and begin the process of self-healing.

SUMMARY

6.00–7.00: Awake; dream diary; breathing exercise; cup of St John's wort tea; hydrotherapy; quiet time; read through Daily Programme Guide

7.00–8.00: Prepare and eat breakfast; prepare packed lunch if necessary

Mid-morning: Cup of St John's wort tea

Lunchtime: Lunch, followed by short walk

Mid-afternoon: Cup of St John's wort tea

Late afternoon: 15 minute quiet time; read dinner menu

Dinnertime: Prepare and eat dinner

8.00–9.00: One hour health workshop – Self-massage

9.45: Quiet time; review of the day

10.00: To bed

Note: Remember to do the extra shopping, listed on page 31, today.

STEP BY STEP

The moment you wake up, write down everything you can remember about the dreams you had last night. Then, before you get out of bed, take three long, slow, deep breaths in and out. Lie still for a moment, breathing quietly. Get up slowly and make yourself a cup of St John's wort tea: 1 tsp of dried flowering tops to a cup of boiling water; brew for a few minutes, strain if necessary. If you need to turn on a heater to make your bathroom warm, do that while the tea is brewing.

After your tea, go to the bathroom, have your normal wash and then do the following hydrotherapy exercise, an indoor version of 'dewy grass walking'. You will need a bathtub or a large bowl and a towel, and should wear a warm tracksuit or dressing gown. If you have a good sense of balance and a bathtub, use Method One below. If you are not so sure on your feet, or you don't have a bathtub, use Method Two.

Method One

Fill the bath half full with cold water. Take off your trousers or pull up your dressing-gown, step into the bath and stand still for a moment. Start walking on the spot, as if you were treading grapes, taking up to 100 steps depending on your general level of fitness. Get out of the bath, sit down and dry your lower legs and feet thoroughly. Get dressed, go into your quiet space and lie down and relax for fifteen minutes.

Method Two

Sit on a chair in the bathroom (or on the toilet with the cover down if more convenient) with a big bowl (or bucket) half full of cold water in front of you. Put both feet in the water then stamp gently up and down, up to 100 times depending on your general level of fitness. Take your feet out of the water and dry your lower legs and feet thoroughly. Get dressed, go into your quiet space and lie down and relax for fifteen minutes.

This hydrotherapy technique is a simple way of stimulating the circulation to the whole body which also benefits the feet and ankles. As you lie and rest, your feet will feel warm and tingly and a general feeling of relaxation will spread through your body.

While you are lying down relaxing, read the following Thought for the Day.

Thought for the Day

To wait for illness to develop before remedying it is to wait until one is thirsty before digging the well.

NEIJING SUWEN

φ

Get up slowly, have a stretch then take your dream diary and mark the different parts with coloured pencil or pen in the same way as yesterday – red for remnants, yellow for things on your mind, green for messages from your subconscious, blue for recurring themes, purple for the apparently unexplainable. After three or four days of doing this you will be able to look at your dream diary in a new and interesting way, reading through each colour separately. You will then begin to see how dreams allow you to communicate with parts of yourself that are not so easily accessible in the noise of the day, and you may even find some useful new ideas and guidance.

Finally, have a look through the rest of this Daily Programme Guide, concentrating on the breakfast and lunch menus. When you have collected your thoughts, leave your quiet space and make breakfast.

7.00–8.00am: Breakfast (plus prepare lunch if necessary)

Breakfast Menu 1 glass unsweetened fruit juice or spring water • fresh fruit salad

> *You will need (per person):*
> 1 apple, cored and chopped
> ½ grapefruit, cut into segments

1 banana, sliced
4–5 dates, stoned and chopped
5 tbs unsweetened fruit juice

Mix all the fruit salad ingredients together in a bowl and serve.

⚘ Health Notes

It could be said that there are only two sorts of medicine in the world, 'conventional' allopathic and traditional naturopathic. Allopathic medicine works on the principle that life is a war with disease as the enemy, an enemy that may strike or invade us at any time and which must be attacked and destroyed with the strongest weapons available. It focuses its resources on disease treatment rather than on health promotion, and its success is measured in terms of more sick people being treated, not less people getting ill in the first place. Naturopathy is the art of inner resource management, a personal way of achieving sustainable health by encouraging what works instead of attacking what doesn't. It involves putting example before explanation, health before disease, prevention before intervention and education before treatment. By putting the emphasis on the basics of health, it allows anyone to become an alchemist – turning the base metal of old patterns into the gold of vitality.

After you have finished your breakfast, sit quietly for a few minutes before doing anything else.

If you need to prepare a packed lunch, refer to the recipe below (page 82). Remember to take some St John's wort tea, some fresh or dried fruit and some bottled water if necessary.

Mid-morning break

A cup of St John's wort tea. If you feel hungry, have some fruit.

Lunchtime

Lunch Menu Avocado and Grapefruit Salad • Carrot Salad •
Mixed Green Salad

You will need (per person):
For the avocado and grapefruit salad:
½ ripe avocado, cut in chunks
¼ grapefruit, cut in chunks
handful watercress, chopped (or, if not available, 3 radishes sliced thinly)
3–4 leaves iceberg lettuce, shredded

For the carrot salad:
1–2 carrots, grated
1 tbs dessicated coconut
2–3 dates, chopped
1–2 tbs lemon juice

For the mixed green salad:
1 handful of spinach or sorrel leaves, chopped
¼ cucumber, cut in chunks
½ celery stalk, chopped
2 tbs sprouts (any type, e.g. beansprouts, alfalfa, mung bean)

Mix the ingredients for each salad, and serve with French dressing.

⚛ **Health Notes**

Avocado is a good source of vitamin B6 and pantothenic acid (the
'anti-stress' vitamin) as well as containing vitamin E, biotin, other B-
group vitamins, potassium, magnesium and zinc. Grapefruit is a source
of potassium as well as calcium, vitamin B3, folate, pantothenic acid,
biotin and, of course, vitamin C. Lettuce contains folic acid and fibre,
watercress provides calcium, iron, zinc, manganese, vitamins A, C, E,
B1, B2, B3 and B6 – and, like other green leaves, both lettuce and
watercress are good sources of essential fatty acids. (A salad dressing

---

made with safflower oil also provides essential fatty acids.) Carrots are rich in antioxidant vitamin A, and both sprouts and spinach contain a whole range of vitamins, minerals and trace elements (including calcium, magnesium, iron and zinc) as well as protein, complex carbohydrate and fibre.

After lunch, sit quietly for five minutes before taking your midday walk. As you walk, notice the colour of the sky and the shapes of any clouds passing overhead as a way of relaxing your eyes and quietening your thoughts.

Mid-afternoon break

A cup of St John's wort tea (plus a piece of fresh fruit if you feel hungry).

Late afternoon

Spend fifteen minutes in your quiet space, sitting or lying down quietly. Take a glass of water, unsweetened fruit juice or vegetable juice with you if you feel thirsty. Before leaving your quiet space, read through the dinner recipe below.

Dinnertime

Dinner Menu   Celeriac and beetroot salad • Herb Salad • Fruit salad

You will need (per person):

For the celeriac and beetroot salad:
2 carrots, grated
¼ small celeriac, grated
½–1 raw beetroot, grated
1 tbs lemon juice

For the herb salad:

1 tbs of each of the following fresh herbs (as available), chopped: mint, parsley, coriander leaf, sorrel (use spinach if sorrel not available)

½ spring onion, sliced

¼ cucumber, sliced

4–5 lettuce leaves, shredded

½ avocado, cubed

1 clove garlic, finely chopped

Mix the ingredients of each salad and serve with French dressing to taste.

For dessert you will need (per person):

1 banana, sliced

1 apple, cored and chopped

10 grapes, halved

1 orange, peeled and chopped

2 fresh apricots, stoned and chopped (or 4 dried apricots)

Mix all the ingredients in a bowl. Sprinkle with some unsweetened fruit juice and a little maple syrup to taste. Serve.

⫸ **Health Notes**

The term 'healing crisis' sounds alarming, but is simply a label for the common experience of illness getting a little worse just before it gets very much better. The symptoms of healing crisis are caused by the higher levels of waste material in the bloodstream that result from a change to a healthier diet. They include mild depression, irritability, vague aches and pains, bad taste in the mouth, slight nausea, more concentrated urine and loose bowels. Strong healing crises are usually only experienced during total fasts or intensive nature cure regimes, but you may be experiencing an exaggerated sense of tiredness as your body mounts a 'clean-up operation'. This is quite normal, and is a sign that the healing process is properly underway.

Sit quietly for a few minutes after your meal before clearing and washing up.

8.00–9.00pm

Health Workshop 4 · SELF-MASSAGE

In this workshop you will learn a simple but powerful self-massage sequence to relax your body and re-balance your natural energy system. It will help you to disperse the energy blocks that lie at the root of many stress-related conditions – tension headaches, stiff neck, cold feet, indigestion, low back pain, etc. – and will allow you to 'ground' any excess or stale energy you may be carrying.

Before you start, make sure your chosen workspace is warm and cosy. You will need two thick towels – one to lie on and the other to put around your shoulders to prevent you from getting cold. If you are going to work on the floor, you will need a rug or mat underneath the towel.

Make up a massage oil as follows: pour 1 tablespoon of today's oil, calendula, into a saucer and then add 2 drops of eucalyptus, 5 drops of marjoram and 1 drop of pine oil. For the parts of the massage sequence that require oil, keep your hands reasonably oily. Each time you put some more oil on to your hands, rub them together for a few seconds to warm the oil before touching your skin. If you run out of oil at any point, just make up a new mixture. If you have any left over at the end, discard it. It is best to make up massage oil fresh whenever possible.

Preparation (no oil)

Take off any watch or jewellery you may be wearing and remove your clothes (at least down to your underwear). If you wear contact lenses, remove these too. Put a towel around your shoulders, sit down and let your mind quieten down for a minute. Let your attention wander around your body, noting which parts feel tense or relaxed, warm or cold, painful or at ease. Take four deep breaths

– in through your nose, out through your mouth – and imagine tension, stress and tiredness leaving your body with each out breath, and being replaced with a peaceful, vital energy on each in breath.

Open your eyes and have a stretch.

Focusing (no oil)

1 Bend your elbows so that your fingertips rest on your shoulders – left hand on left shoulder, right hand on right shoulder.

2 Draw your elbows up in front of your face, then outwards, backwards and down in a circle.

3 Repeat, but this time move your elbows outwards then upwards, inwards and down again in a circle.

4 Hold your arms out in front of you, let your hands hang down loose and shake your wrists gently.

5 Holding your arms still, waggle your hands up and down a few times.

6 Rub your hands together, squeezing each hand with the other and rubbing and squeezing your palms and fingers.

7 Hold your hands up in front of your heart, palms together. Press one hand against the other for a few seconds, then relax.

8 Keep your fingers touching, but move your palms apart. Press your fingers together for a few seconds, then relax.

Head and face (no oil)

1 Rub your palms together and then lightly run them up over your face and down the back of your head several times in a gentle, flowing movement.

2 Cover your face with your hands and run them firmly downwards and outwards over your cheeks and jaw, then around your neck until your fingers meet at the back.

3 Place your thumbs in the corners of your eyes, just by the bridge of your nose. Press upwards lightly and move your thumbs outwards (following the bony ridge above the eye socket) while your forefingers follow the shape of your eyebrows. Repeat.

4 Place your middle fingers underneath your eyes in the inner corners. Press lightly and move your fingers outwards along the bony ridge below the eye socket. Repeat.

5 Place your middle fingers at the inner corner of your eyes again and, applying gentle pressure, glide them downwards and outwards following the contour of your cheekbones and ending up over your jaw muscles. Repeat

6 Hold your fingers over your jaw muscles and massage them gently for a few seconds, using a circular motion.

7 Let your fingertips meet in the middle of your forehead, just above your nose, palms facing inwards. Press your forehead firmly but gently with your fingertips for a few seconds, and then release. Move your fingers upwards a little, press again then release. Continue like this, moving upwards little by little, following the midline of your scalp right over the top of your head and down the back of your neck.

8 Put your fingertips together again on top of your head, just above the hairline. Press your scalp firmly but gently for a few seconds, then release. Move your fingertips gradually apart and downwards, pressing and releasing, until you reach your ears.

9 Put your fingertips on the top of your head again, but now with your hands a couple of inches apart. Work your way backwards, pressing and releasing, ending up on the back of your neck just behind your ears.

10 Rub the palms of your hands together and then move them up over your face, over the top of your head, down the back of your neck. Relax for a minute.

Neck and shoulders (with oil)

1 Turn your head to the right. Place the fingers of your left hand behind your right ear. Gently massage the muscle that runs from there down to your shoulder using a gentle circular motion of your fingers.

2 Do the same on the other side.

3 Place your hands on the back of your neck with fingers about a centimetre apart. Massage the muscles on each side of your spine down your neck to your back.

4 Repeat, but this time with your fingers two centimeteres apart.

5 Put your fingers together at the bottom of your scalp at the back. Massage outwards under the bony ridge that marks the bottom of your skull, until you get to your ears.

6 Support your right elbow in your left hand and place your right hand around the back of your neck from the left. Massage the back of your neck, using all your fingers, moving gradually outwards over the top of your left shoulder. When you get to the shoulder tip, squeeze the muscle that covers it between your fingers and palm.

7 Work back towards the middle, following your shoulderblade inwards and downwards until you get to the spine. Then work upwards, massaging the muscles that lie between your shoulderblade and your spine.

8 Cup your right hand around your left shoulder and massage the muscles at the back of the shoulder. Then move your fingers around the outside to the front, massaging in small circles. Massage the muscles at the front of your shoulder.

Repeat numbers 6 to 8, but this time using your left hand to massage your right neck and shoulder, supporting your left elbow with your right hand.

Arms (with oil)

1 Raise your left arm slightly. Place your right hand flat on your chest with your fingers opposite your left armpit. Massage the muscle that forms the front of your armpit with small circular movements of your fingers.

2 Keeping your thumb at the front, use your fingers to massage the back of your left armpit in the same way.

3 Sit down and rest your left arm on your left thigh, palm facing upwards. Massage the inside of your left arm with your right hand, squeezing with your whole hand (thumb underneath and fingers above), working down from the armpit all the way to the wrist.

4 Put your right palm flat over your left wrist then work your way back up the outside of the left arm, squeezing and releasing until you get to the back of your shoulder.

Repeat numbers 1 to 4, but this time using your left hand to massage the inside and outside of your right arm.

Wrist and hand (with oil)

1 Take your left wrist in your right hand, the back of both hands facing up. Squeeze your wrist for a moment then release.

2 Move your right hand down over the back of your left hand and squeeze again, gently pulling on your wrist.

3 Move your right hand a little further towards your fingers and squeeze again. Carry on like this until you reach your left fingertips.

4 Turn your left palm upwards and massage in between the fingers by squeezing gently with your right thumb and forefinger.

5 Massage the palm of your left hand with your right thumb using small circular movements, making sure you cover the whole area.

6 Now massage each finger on your left hand in turn, starting with the thumb, squeezing, rubbing and pulling each finger gently from base to tip.

7 Repeat numbers 1 to 6, but this time using your left hand to massage your right wrist, palm and fingers.

8 Shake both wrists for a few moments, then make fists and move your hands around in small circles at the wrist. Open your hands, shake your arms briefly then relax.

Chest and Abdomen (with oil)

1 Lie down on your back with your knees bent. Starting at the throat, massage your chest with a flat hand. Work slowly down the middle over your heart until your reach the solar plexus.

2 Keeping your hand flat, massage your abdomen with small circular movements of the fingers, working clockwise around the outside and then gradually inwards in a decreasing spiral, ending up just over your pubic bone. Now put one hand on top of the other, close your eyes and relax for a little while.

3 Stretch both arms out over your head and stretch your legs out too, making yourself as long as possible for a few seconds. Relax.

Back (with oil)

1 Stand up slowly and place your fingers around your middle back, thumbs at your sides, as high up under your arms as you can reach.

2 Massage the muscles on each side of your spine with your fingers.

3 Carry on massaging as you move your hands down your back towards your hips.

4 When you reach the bottom of your back, turn your hands around, placing them on your hips. Massage your lower back and top of your hip bones with your thumbs.

5 Turning your hands as necessary, massage over your sacrum (the flat bone at the bottom of your spine) and then your buttocks.

Thighs, Knees, Lower Legs, Ankles and Feet
(with oil)

1 Sit comfortably on the floor (supporting your back against the wall if necessary) with your legs stretched out in front of you.

2 Bend your left leg a little. Hold your left hand over your left hip and your right hand over the top of your left thigh.

3 Massage the outside and front of your thigh by squeezing and releasing your hands and moving them down your thigh a little at a time.

4 When you reach the knee, put your left hand behind it and the right in front and massage the back and front of your knee.

5 Move your hands to the inside of your thigh and work your way back up to your groin, squeezing and releasing as before.

6 Let your fingers meet around the back of your thigh at the top, then massage down the back of your thigh.

7 Massage the back of your knee again using both hands.

8 Bending your knee as necessary, massage down your lower leg with your fingers behind and thumbs in front, squeezing the lower leg muscles all the way down to the ankle.

9 At the ankle, massage around the joint making small circles with your fingertips.

10 Continue massaging with both hands out over the top of your foot towards your toes.

11 When you reach the toes, give each one a good squeeze and a pull, starting with the little toe and finishing with your big toe.

12 Turn the underside of your foot towards you and massage the sole firmly, starting at the toes and working towards the heel.

13 Straighten your leg out again and move your ankle around in circles a few times, first one way, then the other.

14 Spread your toes out and wiggle them up and down a few times.

15 Repeat numbers 1 to 15 but this time massage your right leg.

Now you have massaged your whole body, you should lie down on your back with a blanket over you and relax for a little while.

φ

Before finishing this health workshop, read throught the notes below about today's herb and oil, and then look through the 'Preparing for Tomorrow' section.

Today's Herb • ST JOHN'S WORT

St John's wort – *Hypericum perforatum* – has been used for healing since ancient times. It is sometimes called 'wound herb', and the name Hypericum comes from a Greek word meaning 'to drive away evil spirits'. Its warming and reassuring qualities make it an ideal support during healing crises, and its restorative effects on the nervous system encourage the process of convalescence and the raising of natural vitality. As an astringent and anti-inflammatory, St John's wort can be used to treat diarrhoea, gastritis, stomach ulcers and arthritis, and its relaxing properties make it an important remedy for headaches, insomnia, depression, anxiety and other nervous problems. It is also a mild local anaesthetic and can be used to ease the discomfort of minor cuts and bruises.

Today's Oil • MARIGOLD (*Calendula officinalis*)

A native of Egypt and the Mediterranean, marigold is another wound-healing herb and an excellent antiseptic and anti-inflammatory remedy for cuts, sores, boils, ulcers and skin problems. It is also a natural antibiotic which can be used to treat herpes simple and to prevent wound infection. Soaking marigold flowers in vegetable oil for a few weeks (preferably in the sun) produces a beautiful deep sunshine-yellow oil which makes a good base for mixing with other essential oils for massage, comfort and healing.

φ

PREPARING FOR TOMORROW

Tomorrow is a special day in *Ten Days To Better Health*, a day of complete rest. Although the Daily Programme Guide contains the usual elements, you should get up when you want and spend as much of the day as possible sleeping, snoozing or just relaxing quietly. The more silent you can be the better, and you should talk as little as possible to others – preferably not at all. Don't forget to have your dream diary by the bed to fill in when you wake up.

9.45–10.00pm

Before going to bed, go into your quiet space and sit quiet and relaxed. Breathe deeply in and out a couple of times, and then review the day's events as usual. When you have finished, half close your eyes and imagine yourself surrounded by a gentle golden light. Then see the light gradually filling your body from head to toe, until you yourself become a source of light, shining outwards with a soft and gentle glow. Remember that healing is not a passive experience – it is an opening of the inner self to a flow of light and love.

Sleep well.

RESTING

On the fifth day, there is a need for complete rest.

SUMMARY

❧

There is no set schedule for today. The object is for you to rest your mind and body as completely as possible, so you should spend as much time as you want just dozing and relaxing. Fill in your dream diary when you first wake up, and then go back to sleep if you want. When you feel like getting up, go through the Morning Sequence below and then spend the rest of the day as quietly as possible, snoozing whenever you feel like it and speaking as little as possible. It is best not to watch TV or listen to the radio, but listening to gentle music is fine. Try and get out for a walk sometime in the afternoon, and do the Health Workshop as usual between 8.00 and 9.00pm so that you can get to bed before 10.00pm. As a way of resting your digestion, the suggested meals consist of fruit only, and you should take them when you feel hungry. Don't forget to drink three cups of today's herb tea (chamomile) during the day, and to drink fresh water whenever you feel thirsty.

MORNING SEQUENCE

Make yourself a cup of chamomile tea (1 teabag, or 1 or 2 tea-spoons of fresh or dried flowers, to a cup of boiling water; brew for a few minutes, strain if necessary), then go into your quiet space and drink it slowly, letting your mind wander where it will. Mark up your dream diary with coloured pencils as usual, then go through the following short self-massage sequence taken from last night's health workshop. Again, remove contact lenses if you wear them.

(Massage oil is *not* required.)

1 Hold your arms out in front of you, let your hands hang down loose and shake your wrists gently.

2 Holding your arms still, waggle your hands up and down a few times.

3 Rub your hands together, squeezing each hand with the other and rubbing and squeezing your palms and fingers.

4 Hold your hands up in front of your heart, palms and fingers touching. Press one hand against the other for a few seconds, then relax.

5 Keep your fingers touching, but move your palms apart. Press your fingers together for a few seconds, then relax.

6 Rub your palms together and then lightly run them up over your face and down the back of your head several times in a gentle, flowing movement.

7 Cover your face with your hands and run them firmly downwards and outwards over your cheeks and jaw, then around your neck until your fingers meet at the back.

8 Place your thumbs in the corners of your eyes, just by the bridge of your nose. Press upwards lightly and move your thumbs outwards (following the bony ridge above the eye socket) while your forefingers follow the shape of your eyebrows. Repeat.

9 Place your middle fingers underneath your eyes in the inner corners. Press lightly and move your fingers outwards along the bony ridge below the eye socket (contact lens wearers beware again!). Repeat.

10 Place your middle fingers at the inner corner of your eyes again and, applying gentle pressure, glide them downwards and outwards following the contour of your cheek bones and ending up over your jaw muscles. Repeat.

11 Hold your fingers over your jaw muscles and massage them gently for a few seconds using a circular motion.

12 Let your fingertips meet in the middle of your forehead, just above your nose, palms facing inwards. Press your forehead firmly but gently with your fingertips for a few seconds, and then release. Move your fingers upwards a little, press again then release. Continue like this, moving upwards little by little, following the midline of your scalp right over the top of your head and down the back of your neck.

13 Put your fingertips together again on top of your head, just above the hairline. Press your scalp firmly but gently for a few seconds, then release. Move your fingertips gradually apart and downwards, pressing and releasing, until you reach your ears.

14 Put your fingertips on the top of your head again, but now with your hands a couple of inches apart. Work your way backwards, pressing and releasing, ending up on the back of your neck just behind your ears.

15 Rub the palms of your hands together and move them up over your face, over the top of your head, down the back of your neck. Relax.

Now read through the Thought for the Day below, and spend a few minutes sitting quietly before leaving your quiet space and having a warm bath or shower. If you are having a bath, add 5 drops of lavender essential oil diluted in 1 tsp sweet almond oil to the water just before you step in. If you prefer a shower, dilute 5 drops of lavender oil in 2 tsp of sweet almond oil and rub it on to your skin after showering.

Thought for the Day

Retreat, to the Western mind, sounds like defeat, but in the eyes of ancient masters withdrawal from the heat of battle was regarded as a major strategic weapon in the armoury of war. People today feel that life is a war fought in the arena of materialism, and to retreat from this for a while is in no sense a defeat. To withdraw into a safe space allows perspective. It gives an understanding of the pattern of life and one's own relationship to it. It helps the mind to reconnect with the body, and the spirit to reconnect with the healing power of nature. Release from the tyranny of time allows understanding of our true self to emerge, as a flower opening its petals to the Sun. Reawakening of consciousness cannot take place within the daily routine of making and taking. It requires freedom, space, quiet, and a willingness to face the accumulated turmoil stored up in the mind.

THE PHI BOOK

φ

Fresh Fruit Breakfast

You will need (per person):
1 banana, sliced
1 pear, cored and sliced
1 apple, cored and sliced
1 portion of another seasonal fresh fruit or berry (e.g. apricot, peach, nectarine, pineapple, plum, cherry, raspberry, strawberry, blackcurrant)
10 grapes, halved
5 tbs unsweetened fruit juice
1 medium glass unsweetened fruit juice or spring water

Mix all the fruit salad ingredients in a bowl and serve.

Fresh Fruit Lunch

To start:

½ paw paw (papaya) or ¼ melon

To follow:

1 banana sliced

1 thick slice pineapple, chopped in chunks

1 apple, cored and sliced

1 pear, cored and sliced

6 grapes, halved

1 portion of another seasonal fresh fruit or berry

5 tbs unsweetened fruit juice

Mix all the fruit salad ingredients in a bowl and serve.

Fresh Fruit Dinner

To start:

½ paw paw (papaya) or ¼ melon

To follow:

1 mango, plus a selection of your favourite fresh fruits and berries

---

⁂ **Health Notes**

Research has shown clearly that eating fresh fruit daily greatly reduces the risk of suffering from heart attack and stroke, as well as cancer. What is more, the beneficial effects of fruit on health seem to depend on eating whole fresh fruit rather than supplements of isolated vitamins or minerals. For example, eating foods rich in the antioxidant beta-carotene is known to be beneficial to health, but research has shown little or no benefit from taking beta-carotene supplements. Unfortunately, the industrialization of agriculture during this century has caused a disproportionate rise in meat and dairy consumption at the expense of fresh fruit and vegetables, particularly in Britain and the

United States – to the extent that many of us now eat only half the recommended daily amount of fresh plant produce. Reversing this trend is one of the major millenial health challenges facing individuals, health care practitioners, farmers and governments.

φ

Health Workshop 5 · RELAXATION

Before you start tonight's workshop, place a thick blanket or a mat on the floor to lie on, and have another blanket to hand to cover you if you feel cold at any point. Lie as flat as you can but make yourself comfortable – you may need a small pillow for your head and perhaps another one under your knees. In this gentle sequence, the periods of relaxation should be longer than the periods of tension.

1 Lie down on your back with your feet apart and pointing outwards, arms by your sides a little out from your body and palms turned upwards.

2 Lift up your right leg tensing the leg and foot muscles as hard as you can. Remember to breathe.

3 Let the tension go and let the leg fall to the floor as you breathe out with a deep sigh. Lie still and feel how tense or relaxed the leg muscles are now.

4 Lift up your right leg again, this time spreading your toes as much as you can. Let go with a deep sigh. Lie still with your right leg relaxed and notice how it feels different from the left leg.

5 Lift up your left leg, tensing the leg and foot muscles as hard as you can. Remember to breathe.

6 Let the tension go and let the leg fall to the floor as you breathe out with a deep sigh. Lie still and feel how tense or relaxed the leg muscles are now.

7 Lift up your left leg again, this time spreading your toes as much as you can. Let go with a deep sigh. Lie still and notice how both your legs feel now.

8 Now tense your bottom muscles as hard as you can, then let go and relax.

9 Arch your back and lift it off the floor while keeping your bottom and shoulders touching the floor. Relax and lie still.

10 Breathe out, emptying your lungs as completely as possible and at the same time push your back down on to the floor. Relax.

11 Lift your right arm up, tensing the muscles and making a tight fist. Remember to breathe. Let the arm fall, and relax.

12 Lift up your right arm again, tensing the muscles but this time spreading your fingers as wide as possible. Let the arm fall, relax and feel the difference between your right and left arms.

13 Lift your left arm up, tensing the muscles and making a tight fist. Remember to breathe. Let the arm fall, and relax.

14 Lift up your left arm again, tensing the muscles but this time spreading your fingers as wide as possible. Let the arm fall, relax and see how both arms feel now.

15 Push your shoulders down on to the floor keeping your arms relaxed. Let go and lie still.

16 Lift your shoulders up off the floor without lifting your head. Relax.

17 Pull your shoulders up around your ears as far as you can. Let go and relax.

18 Push your shoulders downwards towards your feet as hard as you can. Remember to breathe. Lie still and see how your shoulders feel now.

19 Arch your neck by looking behind you as far as you can (like looking above you if you were standing). Relax again.

20 Lift your head forward towards your chest. Let go and lie still.

21 Clench your teeth and press your tongue against the roof of your mouth. Relax.

22 Yawn, opening your mouth as wide as you can. Close it again.

23 Screw your eyes up tight. Relax.

24 Make a deep frown on your forehead. Relax and notice how your head and face feel.

25 Finally, think about each part of your body in turn – starting at the feet and working up through legs, bottom, back, arms, shoulders, neck and face – letting each part feel as heavy as possible, as if sinking into the floor. Then lie still for a little while without thinking about anything in particular.

26 Before you get up slowly, have a good stretch and a yawn.

φ

Before finishing this health workshop, read through the notes below about today's herb and oil, and then look through the 'Preparing for Tomorrow' section.

Today's Herb · CHAMOMILE *(Matricaria recutita)*

Chamomile is a gentle healer which promotes relaxation and repair, calming the nerves and stimulating the immune system. It is a gentle sedative with a profoundly soothing effect on the mind and nervous system, and is especially helpful for resolving bottled-up tension and anger as well as anxiety, restlessness, impatience and sleeplessness. It can also be used to help heal inflammation – external and internal – and is an effective way of relieving indigestion. Its gentleness and wide range of uses makes chamomile particularly suitable for children.

Today's Oil · LAVENDER *(Lavendula officinalis)*

Lavender is a native of the Mediterranean region, with a name that comes from the Latin word meaning 'to wash'. It is a sweet smelling and powerful antiseptic with an old reputation for healing grief and pain, and is a fine remedy for dealing with stress and nervous tension. A bath or foot bath with lavender oil is refreshing, relaxing and heart-warming, and is especially beneficial in the evening to encourage a good night's sleep. It also helps the body to deal with infection and can be used in the treatment of skin conditions like acne and eczema. As a mild pain-killer, lavender oil can be used to ease neuralgic, rheumatic and arthritic aches and pains, and is an excellent first-aid remedy for insect bites (applied neat).

φ

PREPARING FOR TOMORROW

Tomorrow you will be using the herb nettle and the essential oil rosemary. Breakfast will be a fresh fruit salad, lunch a mixed salad and dinner guacamole with vegetable sticks. From this point until the end of the programme your meals will get gradually fuller and more varied as your vitality increases. Set your alarm tonight for 6.00am (or two hours before you leave for work or start your normal daily activities). Remember to have your dream diary and a pen by the bed for when you wake up. Day Six – REVIEWING will start with your dream diary, a breathing exercise, a cup of nettle tea and a morning quiet time including a relaxation sequence.

Before going to bed, go into your quiet space and sit relaxed. Breathe deeply in and out a couple of times, and then review the day's events as usual. When you have finished, read through the following passage and spend a few minutes reflecting on its meaning before going to bed.

Thirty spokes unite at the centre
And because of the part where nothing exists
We have the use of the wheel.

Clay is moulded into pots
And because of the space where nothing exists
We are able to use them as vessels.

Doors and windows are cut in the walls of a house
And because of the empty space
We are able to use them.

Thus while we have the benefit of existence,
We are constantly making use of non-existence.

LAO TSU

Sleep well.

REVIEWING

On the sixth day, there is a review of the past, and of the influences and experiences that have shaped your life and your personality.

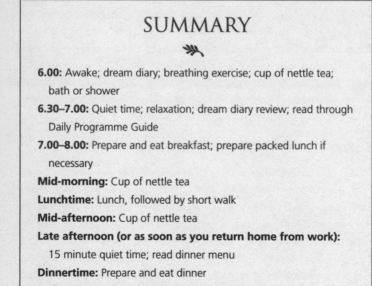

SUMMARY

6.00: Awake; dream diary; breathing exercise; cup of nettle tea; bath or shower

6.30–7.00: Quiet time; relaxation; dream diary review; read through Daily Programme Guide

7.00–8.00: Prepare and eat breakfast; prepare packed lunch if necessary

Mid-morning: Cup of nettle tea

Lunchtime: Lunch, followed by short walk

Mid-afternoon: Cup of nettle tea

Late afternoon (or as soon as you return home from work): 15 minute quiet time; read dinner menu

Dinnertime: Prepare and eat dinner

8.00–9.00: One hour health workshop – Self Audit

9.45: Quiet time; review of the day

10.00: To bed

STEP BY STEP

6.00am

The moment you wake up, write down everything you can remember about the dreams you had last night. Then, before you get out of bed, take three deep breaths. Count up to nine in your head as you breathe in, and back down again to one as you breathe out. Leave a count of three between each breath, and remember to push your tummy outwards on the in breath to encourage the diaphragm to fill your lungs from the bottom up. Lie still for a moment or two, breathing quietly.

Get up slowly, have a stretch and a yawn, and make yourself a cup of nettle tea – 1 tsp dried herb or one teabag to a cup of boiling water; brew for a few minutes, strain if necessary. After your tea, use the bathroom and have a warm bath or shower. If you are having a bath, add 5 drops of rosemary essential oil mixed with 1 tsp sweet almond oil to the water. If you prefer a shower, dilute 5 drops of rosemary oil in 2 tsp of sweet almond oil, and rub into your skin after your shower.

6.30am

When you have washed and dressed, go into your quiet space, light a candle and sit quietly for five minutes. Then lie down and think about each part of your body in turn – starting at the feet and working up through legs, bottom, back, arms, shoulders, neck and face – letting each part feel as heavy as possible, as if sinking into the floor. Lie still for a minute without thinking about anything in particular, then repeat the exercise. Still lying relaxed, read the following Thought for the Day. Then have a good stretch and a yawn and get up slowly.

Thought for the Day

Even though you tie a hundred knots, the string remains one.

Rumi

φ

Take your dream diary and mark it up as usual in different colours. Then spend ten minutes reading through the diary from the beginning, colour by colour – i.e. read all the entries marked in red for remnants, then those in yellow for things on your mind, green for messages from your subconscious, blue for recurring themes and purple for the apparently unexplainable. Pay particular attention to the entries you have marked in yellow and green.

Dream interpretation is a fascinating subject, and deciding for yourself which parts of your dreams represent mental housekeeping, which are symptoms of repressed fears and anxieties, and which are trying to give you helpful information is certainly a worthwhile exercise. From the point of view of personal development, the most interesting and important thing about dreams is that they allow you to have a conscious experience of a different type of reality. To put it another way, they give you the sensation of another sort of consciousness, free of your material body. This is why meditation – which also leads to an experience of 'expanded' consciousness – is both restful and good for health. Like dreaming, it provides the mind with a chance to sort itself out and communicate, but has the advantage that you can do it anywhere, anytime, without needing to fall asleep. It is well known that people deprived of 'dream sleep' rapidly become exhausted and disoriented, but people who meditate regularly feel clearer mentally, less tired and more alert. Meditation is the subject of the Health Workshop on Day 8.

As you carry on recording your dreams and reviewing them each day, you will find that they can tell you a great deal about the patterns that govern your life. (One word of caution: making decisions on the basis of dreams is generally to be avoided. It is better to regard them as sources of information which broaden your perspective, and thus help you to make better decisions.)

φ

Have a brief look through the rest of this Daily Programme Guide, concentrating on the breakfast and lunch menus. When you have collected your thoughts, leave your quiet space and make breakfast.

7.00–8.00am: Breakfast (plus prepare lunch if necessary)

Breakfast Menu 1 glass unsweetened fruit juice or spring water • fresh fruit salad

You will need (per person):
1 apple, cored and chopped
½ grapefruit, cut into segments
1 banana, sliced
4–5 dates, stoned and chopped
5 tbs unsweetened fruit juice

Mix all the fruit salad ingredients together in a bowl and serve.

Health Notes

Most people know that organic produce tastes better, is more nutritious and is better for the environment. Unfortunately, as things stand at the moment, cheap, locally grown organic produce is hard to come by for most of us, but there are still many things we can do to hasten the development of a gentler and more sustainable agricultural system. Above all, we should buy fresh, unprocessed produce whenever possible, and go out of our way to choose things grown locally by supporting smallholders, 'box' schemes, farm shops, roadside stalls of keen local gardeners, pick your own, etc. We should also eat seasonally as much as we can, and should find and support local organic growers when practicable. Organic or not, as far as health is concerned the first priority is to eat fresh and in season, and to eat as much plant-based food as possible.

Mid-morning break

A cup of nettle tea. If you feel hungry, have some fresh or dried fruit. If possible, try and find five minutes to repeat the relaxation exercise you did earlier this morning. Though it is easier to do lying down, it can still be quite effective when sitting in a chair (perhaps with your feet up).

Lunchtime

Lunch Menu Mixed salad

You will need (per person):
¼ cucumber, thinly sliced
1 tomato, cut into quarters
1 stalk celery
½ cup sweetcorn
100g/3½oz raw mushrooms, cleaned and sliced
1 handful of lettuce, shredded
1 handful watercress, chopped (optional)
4 or 5 radishes, sliced

Mix all the ingredients and serve with French dressing to taste.
If you feel like it, have a piece of fresh fruit for dessert.

⋙   **Health Notes**

Since the 1950s, 'eat more fibre' has been the catchphrase of the diet and health conscious – and with good reason. Diets rich in natural fibre help prevent several serious diseases such as bowel cancer, diverticulitis, coronary heart disease and gallstones, and are the surest way of avoiding constipation and haemorrhoids. Fibre is not just an indigestible waste product; the body uses different sorts of fibre in several different ways, and it plays an important role in the metabolism of fats and sugars, as well as helping to maintain a healthy environment in our bowels. Fibre – or non-starch polysaccharide as it is now called – is *only*

---

found in plant foods. There is none in meat or dairy products. The fact that the majority of people in the West are constantly on the verge of constipation illustrates the major problem of late twentieth-century diet: we eat too much meat and dairy produce and not enough fresh fruits, vegetables and whole grains.

After lunch, sit quietly for five minutes before taking your midday walk. As you walk, be aware of the different smells and odours around you, and the memories or experiences they bring to mind.

Mid-afternoon break

A cup of nettle tea. If you feel hungry, have some fresh or dried fruit. Again, try and find five minutes to repeat the relaxation exercise you did this morning.

Late afternoon (or as soon as you return home from work):

Spend fifteen minutes in your quiet space, sitting or lying down quietly. Take a glass of water, unsweetened fruit juice or vegetable juice with you if you feel thirsty. Before leaving your quiet space, read through the dinner recipe below:

Dinnertime

Dinner Menu   Guacamole with vegetable sticks

You will need (per person):
1–2 ripe avocado(s)
2 tsp lemon juice
1 small clove garlic, crushed
¼ tsp salt
pinch cayenne pepper (optional)
1 tbs olive oil

¼ teaspoon paprika

1 tbs chopped parsley

Some mixed raw vegetables (e.g. carrot, celery, beetroot, apple, fennel, spring onion), chopped into sticks, plus some cauliflower florets, cucumber chunks, mushrooms, radishes and young green beans – according to taste and availability.

Blend or mash the avocado with the lemon juice, garlic, salt and olive oil, adding a little water if necessary to get a creamy consistency. Garnish with parsley and paprika, then serve as a dip with a generous selection of raw vegetables.

☙ Health Notes

Some of the chemical reactions that enable our bodies to release energy from food also produce by-products known as free radicals which can damage the membranes that surround our body cells. Luckily, our cell membranes contain chemicals called antioxidants which prevent free radicals from doing damage. Since we make our bodies out of the foods we eat, a good intake of antioxidant vitamins and minerals such as vitamin E, vitamin C, beta-carotene and selenium, help to ensure protection against free radicals, and may also be important for avoiding heart disease, cancer and neurological conditions including Parkinson's disease. Since polluted twentieth-century urban air and cigarette smoke also contain free radicals, it is clearly important to make sure that our diet is rich in antioxidants, and the easiest way to do this is to eat vegetables, fruits, nuts, seeds and cold-pressed polyunsaturated vegetable oils.

Sit quietly for a few minutes after your meal before clearing and washing up.

8.00–9.00pm

Health Workshop 6 · SELF AUDIT

There is a saying that each individual is really three people: the person others see, the person we see ourselves, and the person we really are. The purpose of this workshop is to help you get a clearer picture of the person you really are by investigating the influences that have shaped your personality. All you need is a pen and several sheets of paper.

Personality is something we learn – a mixture of attitudes, beliefs, behaviours and responses drawn from our experience of family, education, culture, religion, friends and relationships. Some of the influences that shaped our personalities in the past are not those we would have chosen if we had known then what we know now. For example, parents who are very demanding tend to produce young adults who are both anxious and demanding themselves; religions that emphasize sin can produce believers haunted by guilt; a music teacher who once told you that you sing off key may have produced an adult convinced that they are tone deaf. Given the choice, few people *want* to be anxious, demanding, guilt ridden or tone deaf . . .

This is not about blaming others for the way you are. It is about facing up to the fact that some aspects of who you are are not how you want them to be simply because you have been influenced by the attitudes and expectations of others, at times when you felt you had no choice. If you can identify where the various traits in your personality have their roots, you can – if you like – uproot them. In other words, you can choose to discard those aspects of your personality that are the result of other people's problems, and develop the ones that are the result of your own experiences and inner convictions.

You can be whoever you want to be. You can choose what sort of a personality you use as a vehicle for communicating with the world. You do not have to argue in the same way your parents argued, using the same words. You do not have to share the prejudices of those around you. You do not have to draw the same conclusions as your teachers, and you do not have to base your religious convictions on other people's experience. If you look squarely at the traits that make up your personality, identify where they come from, and weed out the ones that were developed in you by circumstance instead of by your own design, you can be truly yourself. Once you start being yourself, you can go on developing your personality in the light of your own experience, and will be entirely responsible for the person you are.

Take your pen and paper and make nine lists (each containing at least five items) as follows:

1. People who have influenced your life (including authors of books that are important to you)
2. Places that have influenced your life
3. Particular dates, times or events that have influenced your life
4. Your positive personality traits
5. Your negative personality traits
6. Things you find a comfort in life
7. Things that have caused sadness in your life
8. Things that give you satisfaction
9. Things which you fear

To complete the 'influence' lists, let your mind drift back over your life, adding items to the different lists as the memories come up. Don't think too hard when filling in the other lists. Write what comes to mind, moving back and forth from list to list as things occur to you.

When the lists are complete, look through them a few times and try to identify which influences produced which personality traits. If you have time, see also if you can relate any of your personality traits to your comforts, sadnesses, satisfactions and fears. (If other memories come up while you are doing this, add to the appropriate lists as necessary.) Then draw a circle around all the personality traits that form a part of who you really want to be, and strike through with a line (/) those you would like to discard. Keep these lists for tomorrow night's workshop.

φ

Before leaving this workshop, read through the notes below about today's herb and oil, and then look through the 'Preparing for Tomorrow' section.

Today's Herb • NETTLE (Urtica dioica)

Nettle is one of the world's most common and misunderstood weeds. Depite its reputation as a plant to be wary of, it is a tasty, nutritious vegetable (when boiled, the sting disappears entirely) and a useful medicine. Nettle tea has been used for centuries as a blood purifier and 'spring cleanser', and since it is rich in nutrients it is also an excellent aid to convalescence. In the old herbal tradition, it was regarded as having heating and drying qualities, and an ability to consume cold and moist conditions and add energy to the body. Its modern use as a circulatory stimulant and diuretic reflects this old understanding, and its ability to cleanse the body of accumulated waste makes it particularly useful in the treatment of arthritis and skin conditions.

Today's Oil • ROSEMARY (Rosmarinus officinalis)

Rosemary is a herb of legend, dedicated in ancient times to the Goddess of Love. It symbolizes faithfulness, friendship and remembrance and has a reputation for improving the memory and focusing the mind. Its warming, comforting qualities make it useful for unlocking buried tensions and emotions, making it easier to look at past experiences in order to accept them and let them go. It is also an energizing tonic to the digestion, circulation and nervous system, useful in the treament of arthritis, headache, hair loss, indigestion and wind.

PREPARING FOR TOMORROW

Tomorrow you will be using the herb yarrow and the oil melissa. Breakfast will be fruit salad with fresh and dried fruits, lunch a beetroot, mint and apple salad with a mixed raw vegetable salad, and dinner spicy chickpeas with green beans and potatoes, followed by yoghurt and fruit. (If you are going to use dried chickpeas, they will need to be rinsed and soaked overnight. The recipe requires 50 grams/2oz dry weight.) Set your alarm tonight for 6.00am, or two hours before you leave for work or start your normal daily activities. Day Seven – TRANSFORMING will start with a cup of yarrow tea, some stretching exercises, a bath or shower and morning quiet time.

9.45–10.00pm

Before going to bed, go into your quiet space and sit quiet and relaxed. Breathe deeply in and out a couple of times, then review the day's events as usual. When you have finished, lie down and go through the relaxation sequence that you have been using during the day. Then read through the following brief passage, and spend a few minutes reflecting on its meaning before going to bed.

If you understand how the chains were put on, you can understand how to loosen and escape from them.

THE PHI BOOK

φ

Sleep well.

Tuesday

TRANSFORMING

On the seventh day, you start to transform and let go of those things from the past that separate you from health and peace of mind in the present.

SUMMARY

6.00: Awake; dream diary; stretching; cup of yarrow tea; bath or shower

6.30–7.00: Quiet time; read through Daily Programme Guide

7.00–8.00: Prepare and eat breakfast; prepare packed lunch if necessary

Mid-morning: Cup of yarrow tea

Lunchtime: Lunch, followed by short walk

Mid-afternoon: Cup of yarrow tea

Late afternoon (or as soon as you return home from work): 15 minute quiet time; read dinner menu

Dinnertime: Prepare and eat dinner

8.00–9.00: One hour health workshop – Autosuggestion

9.45: Quiet time; review of the day

10.00: To bed

STEP BY STEP

6.00am

Fill in your Dream Diary as soon as you wake up. When you are ready to get out of bed, stand up and take three slow deep breaths in and out. Relax for a minute, then go through the following stretching sequence, taken from the Health Workshop on Day 2.

1 Stand relaxed, feet slightly apart. Put your hands together palm to palm in front of you, then stretch your arms up over your head (hands still together). Keeping your arms over your head, stretch the muscles on the right side of your body by bending slowly sideways to the left. Then stretch your left side by bending sideways to the right. Let you arms hang down by your sides and relax.

2 Fold your hands behind your back, fingers interlocked, and stretch your arms downwards and away from your back while you lift your chest forwards and up, arching your spine and looking upwards and backwards as far as you can. Then let your hands go, straighten your back and neck, look ahead and relax.

3 Stand with your arms by your sides, feet a little apart. Lower your head very slowly forward until your chin touches your chest, then continue to bend forwards, curving your back slowly and progressively from the top downwards (keeping your lower back straight as long as possible). Your head and arms should hang down loose and heavy as you bend. When your fingertips are at the same level as your knees, unfold yourself by uncurling your back from the bottom upwards, breathing deeply and sighing as you breathe out. Stand upright and relax.

4 Hold your hands up in front of your heart, palms together. As you take a slow deep breath in, lift your arms upwards as far as you can, palms still together. As you breathe out, move your hands apart, outwards and backwards in a big circle, ending up with your palms meeting in front of your heart again. Stand still for a moment, breathing gently.

Now make yourself a cup of yarrow tea – 1 tsp of dried herb or one teabag to a cup of boiling water, brew for a few minutes, strain if necessary. After your tea, use the bathroom and have a warm bath or shower. If you are having a bath, add 2–3 drops of melissa essential oil mixed in 1 tsp of sweet almond oil to the water. If you prefer a shower, dilute 2–3 drops of melissa oil in 2 tsp of sweet almond oil and rub it into your skin after your shower.

6.30am

When you are washed and dressed, go into your quiet space, light a candle and sit quietly for five minutes. Then take your notes from last night's workshop and look through them for a few minutes, adding to the lists if anything else comes to mind. Put them aside and sit quietly for another couple of minutes with your eyes half closed, letting your mind wander where it will. Then read the following Thought for the Day.

Thought for the Day

Our deepest fear is not that we are inadequate
Our deepest fear is that we are powerful beyond measure
It is our light not our darkness that most frightens us
We ask ourselves 'Who am I to be brilliant, gorgeous, talented and
*   fabulous?'*
Actually, who are you not to be?

DESMOND TUTU (attributed)

φ

Have a good stretch and a yawn, then look briefly through the rest of this Daily Programme Guide, concentrating on the breakfast and lunch menus. When you have collected your thoughts, leave your quiet space and make breakfast.

7.00–8.00am: Breakfast (plus prepare lunch if necessary)

Breakfast Menu 1 glass unsweetened fruit juice or spring water • fruit salad with fresh and dried fruits

You will need (per person):

1 thick slice pineapple, chopped

1 banana, sliced

handful of grapes, halved

1 apple, cored and chopped

3–4 dates, stoned and chopped

3–4 dried apricots, stoned and chopped

5 tbs unsweetened fruit juice

Mix all the fruit salad ingredients together in a bowl and serve.

⚜ **Health Notes**

We consume several different types of fat in our diet and many people are not entirely clear about which are good for health and which bad. The facts are: 1. We should eat less saturated fat. 2. We should avoid hydrogenated and trans fats. 3. We should include some polyunsaturated oils in our diet. 4. We should do what we can to decrease our fat intake overall. In practical terms, the easiest way to achieve all this is to increase our fresh fruit and vegetable consumption and decrease our meat and dairy intake. Meat, milk, cheese and eggs are the main dietary sources of saturated fat. We should avoid processed foods containing animal fats or hydrogenated vegetable oils where possible, and use table spreads made of polyunsaturated vegetable oils that contain a minimum of hydrogenated oils and trans fats. (Butter contains about 5 per cent trans fats and is high in saturated fat.) Eating plenty of green leafy vegetables and including some polyunsaturated oils like sunflower or safflower in our diet will ensure a good supply of essential fatty acids.

Mid-morning break

A cup of yarrow tea. If you feel hungry, have some fresh or dried fruit.

Lunchtime

Lunch Menu   Beetroot, mint and apple salad • Mixed raw vegetable salad

> *You will need (per person):*
>
> **For the beetroot salad:**
> 1 small beetroot, grated
> 1 apple, grated
> 1 small handful fresh mint, finely chopped (or 1 tsp dried)
> 2 tbs safflower oil
> 1 tbs lemon juice
> small piece fresh horseradish, grated finely (optional)

Mix the beetroot, apple, mint, oil and lemon juice in a bowl, garnish with horseradish and season to taste.

> **For the mixed raw vegetable salad:**
> ¼ small cauliflower, cut into florets
> 1 carrot, finely sliced
> ¼ cucumber, chopped into chunks
> 1 tomato, quartered
> 1 spring onion, chopped finely
> 5–6 lettuce leaves, shredded
> a few olives (optional)

Mix together the vegetable salad ingredients in another bowl, and garnish with olives. Serve both salads with French Dressing to taste.

If you feel like it, have one or two pieces of fresh fruit for dessert.

⅗⃥ Health Notes

Many people regard cholesterol as a dangerous substance but in fact cholesterol is a normal component of our body cells and necessary for the production of bile and various hormones. The body is able to make all the cholesterol it needs out of the food we eat, so there is no actual need to eat foods that contain cholesterol. If we eat a diet rich in saturated fat (i.e. a diet high in meat and dairy foods) the amount of cholesterol in our bloodstream increases and it is this that puts us at risk of heart disease and stroke from clogged-up arteries. In other words, it is not eating cholesterol itself that is dangerous, it is eating large quantities of foods that contain a lot of cholesterol, because these foods are also high in saturated fat. Plants contain no cholesterol and are naturally rich in polyunsaturated fat, so eating more of them naturally decreases our risk of having too much cholesterol in our blood.

After lunch, sit quietly for five minutes before taking your midday walk. As you walk, try the following simple observation exercise: be aware of the various colours that make up the visual landscape you are walking through, and try and decide which colour predominates and which colours you would have to use if you were painting a picture.

Mid-afternoon break

A cup of yarrow tea. If you feel hungry, have some fresh or dried fruit.

Late afternoon (or as soon as you return home from work):

Spend fifteen minutes in your quiet space, sitting or lying down quietly. Take a glass of water, unsweetened fruit juice or vegetable juice with you if you feel thirsty. Before leaving your quiet space, read through the dinner recipe below.

Dinnertime

Dinner Menu Spicy chickpeas with green beans and potatoes
• yoghurt with fruit

> *You will need:*
> 100g/4oz drained tinned chickpeas (or 50g/2oz dried chickpeas, rinsed,
>   soaked overnight, rinsed again then boiled for an hour before use)
> 2 tbs olive oil
> ½ tsp ground cumin
> ½ tsp ground coriander
> ½ onion, chopped
> 1 clove garlic, finely chopped
> 2 tomatoes (fresh or tinned), chopped
> 1 tbs parsley, finely chopped
> ½ tsp dried thyme
> pinch cayenne pepper (optional)
> ½ tsp fresh grated ginger
> a little water or vegetable stock
> salt to taste

Heat the oil in a large saucepan or wok, add the cumin, coriander, garlic and onion and stir-fry gently for 3 to 4 minutes until the onion is soft. Add the chickpeas, stir, then add the rest of the ingredients. Bring to the boil and simmer gently for 15 minutes, adding a little water from time to time if necessary. Adjust the seasoning to taste before serving.

> *You will also need:*
> 500g/1lb 2oz potatoes, peeled and chopped
> 180g/6oz young green beans, topped and tailed

While the chickpeas are simmering, put the potatoes on to boil and lightly steam the green beans. **Save half the potatoes and beans for lunch tomorrow.**

For dessert:

1 soya yoghurt

1 portion seasonal berries or fruit, finely chopped

〰 Health Notes

If there was a competition for natural super-foods, chickpeas would certainly be a contender for first place. As well as containing about 30 per cent of their calories in the form of protein (more than duck or plaice), they are low in fat, contain no cholesterol and are rich in complex carbohydrates and fibre. They are an excellent source of zinc, iron, manganese and copper and contain significant amounts of calcium, magnesium, potassium, selenium, vitamin E, vitamins B1, B2, B3 and B6, folate and pantothenic acid. They are cheap to buy, easy to prepare and add real body to dishes that include them.

Sit quietly for a few minutes after your meal before clearing and washing up.

8.00pm–9.00pm

Health Workshop 7 · AUTOSUGGESTION

Autosuggestion is a safe, simple and ancient technique for 'programming' the subconscious mind to help us feel how we want to feel, and achieve the things that we want to achieve. In fact it is so simple that many people are not inclined to take it seriously, despite numerous examples in our society of the power of simple suggestion. Think for a moment – what's your favourite TV advert? Your favourite (or least favourite) advertising jingle? Which company has more or less given its name to the vacuum cleaner? What fizzy drink comes in red cans with white lettering? Which fast-food chain uses red and yellow as its main colours? How do you know these things? Because they have been imprinted on your subconscious by repetition. In the end, you have only to glance at a logo, see a particular colour, or hear a tune to think of – and possibly buy – a particular product. The billions of pounds spent each year on advertising are an impressive testament to the idea that you can get people to do things automatically (i.e. buy) by imprinting things on their subconscious. Marketing is all about converting wants into needs, and its objective is to make you part with your resources by imprinting someone else's message on your mind. Autosuggestion is about encouraging your body to be well, your emotions peaceful and your mind calm by imprinting your *own* messages on your subconscious.

If you have tried learning a foreign language (or a complicated physical skill), you will know that repetition is the key to learning by experience. With language, first you listen to people speaking, then you understand what they're saying and finally you speak yourself. With autosuggestion, first you listen to yourself repeating a message until your subconscious understands, then your subconscious organizes your physical, mental and emotional processes to make the content of your suggestion a reality. Perhaps the best known autosuggestion in the Western world is 'Day by day in every way I am getting better and better'. It has its origin in the work of Emile Coué, who had remarkable success in the early part of this century using autosuggestion techniques in the treatment of a whole range of serious physical and mental conditions. His work is not well known these days, but his observations on the process of autosuggestion form the basis of a powerful self-healing method. In fact, affirmations of one sort or another are now used in all sorts of situations, from sport and business to personal and spiritual development.

There are four important rules for the successful use of autosuggestion. First, your self-healing affirmations have to bear some relationship to your current situation. Although autosuggestion is about achieving what you want, starting off with something too grandiose or ambitious usually means that your subconscious will take no notice, because it has no means of bridging the gap between how things are and how you want them to be. So, if you have a chronic illness for example, it is far better to affirm that day by day you will get better and better than to repeat 'I am completely well' to yourself (which, since it is obviously not true, causes discouragement rather than progress).

Second, it is important that autosuggestions start off with a phase like 'Day by day' or 'From this moment on' or 'For every moment that passes' or something similar. This allows for the ups and downs of normal progress and ensures that your subconscious recognizes your affirmation as both true and achievable.

Third, autosuggestion is a dynamic process and your affirmations should change to match your situation as it improves. Suppose you are using autosuggestion to deal with anxiety. If you notice that your anxiety is getting less and only occurs in one or two particular situations, you should adapt your affirmation to focus on these situations. Autosuggestion is about moving forward slowly but surely, without attempting big leaps into change.

Fourth, affirmations have to be positive in order to work. Again, if fear or anxiety is your problem, it doesn't usually help to use autosuggestions like 'Day by day my fear is getting less and less'. It is far more effective to use affirmations that encourage the development of what you want rather than the abolition of what you don't want. With fear, for example, an effective first autosuggestion might be 'Day by day I am feeling more calm and more confident'; for a chronic illness one might try 'Day by day I am becoming stronger and more healthy'.

With these points in mind, you can start to develop your own autosuggestions as a way of encouraging the things that you would like to see happen in your life. Having chosen what you want to affirm, all you have to do is repeat it to yourself 20 times in the morning when you wake up, 20 times in the evening before you go to sleep, and anytime during the day that your mind is 'idling' – journeys, standing in queues, or doing any repetitive task. Each evening when you review the day, consider how much progress has been made and decide whether or not to modify or change your affirmation. With patience and perseverance, you will be amazed how short a time it takes to achieve results.

So now look through your Self Audit notes from last night, and try to identify what is at the root of the dissatisfactions you have with your life. In most cases, it will be one of the following: poor health, lack of resources, fear, anger, guilt, or desire. Try and formulate a short affirmation to help you make a change for the better. Here are some examples to help you:

- **Poor health**: Day by day, in every way, I am getting better and better.

- **Lack of resources**: From this moment on, I accept that I am worthy to receive what I need.

- **Fear and anger**: From this moment on, whatever the circumstances, I feel calm and at peace.

- **Guilt**: From this moment on, I accept forgiveness.

- **Desire**: Day by day I accept what I need with joy, and give what I can with love.

Write down your affirmation together with the date and time, memorize it and then, sitting quiet and relaxed, repeat it to yourself twenty times (either in a quiet voice or in your head, according to preference). Do the same again before going to sleep tonight and again when you wake up tomorrow morning (after filling in your dream diary). Continue repeating your affirmation any time you get a few idle moments during the day, and continue for as many days as it takes to notice a change for the better. If the affirmation ceases to 'ring true', it means that your subconscious has got the message, and you can turn your attention to a new issue and design a new affirmation to deal with it. With practice, you will find that autosuggestion can be used to bring about almost any change you want in your life.

φ

Before leaving this workshop, read through the notes below about today's herb and oil, and then look through the 'Preparing for Tomorrow' section.

Today's Herb · YARROW *(Achillea millefolium)*

In ancient times, yarrow was regarded as a sacred herb, used by the Druids for divination and by Chinese sages for casting the I Ching. During the Middle Ages it was known as a 'heal-all', and it is still much valued by herbalists for its ability to support and stimulate different body systems. It has a particular effect on the circulation, lowering blood pressure and slowing the heart, but can also be used to reduce fevers, treat infection, stimulate the digestion and ease period pain. On a psychological level it brings confidence, and can therefore encourage the letting go of old fears, regrets, attachments and worries.

Today's Oil · LEMON BALM *(Melissa officinalis)*

Melissa is a sweet and cheerful herb, cherished by many cultures over thousands of years. It is said to 'make the heart merry', and has even been called the elixir of life. The oil has a unique uplifting quality which reduces tension, calms a troubled heart and stills a worried mind, making it possible to see life in a new perspective. It is indicated for conditions such as tension headache, migraine, depression, anxiety, high blood pressure, indigestion and asthma, and its anti-viral properties make it useful in the management of herpes simplex infections.

φ

PREPARING FOR TOMORROW

Tomorrow you will be using the herb angelica and the oil frankincense. Breakfast will be muesli with fruits, nuts and seeds, lunch a Catalan salad, and dinner stuffed mushrooms with rice and creamed spinach. Set your alarm tonight for 6.00am, or two hours before you leave for work or start your normal daily activities. Day Eight

– AWAKENING will start with autosuggestion, a cup of angelica tea, some stretching exercises, a bath or shower and morning quiet time.

9.45–10.00pm

Before going to bed, go into your quiet space and sit quiet and relaxed. Breathe deeply in and out a couple of times, then review the day's events as usual. When you have finished, half close your eyes and repeat your new affirmation twenty times. Open your eyes, have a yawn and a stretch and read the following brief passage before going to bed.

> *You must dive deep into the sea to get the pearls.*
> *What good does it do to dabble among the waves near the shore*
> *And to assert that the sea has no pearls?*

SAI BABA

Sleep well.

Wednesday

AWAKENING

On the eighth day, vitality and enthusiasm for life start to increase.

SUMMARY

❧

6.00: Awake; dream diary; autosuggestion; stretching; cup of angelica tea; bath or shower

6.30–7.00: Quiet time; read through Daily Programme Guide

7.00–8.00: Prepare and eat breakfast; prepare packed lunch if necessary

Mid-morning: Cup of angelica tea

Lunchtime: Lunch, followed by short walk

Mid-afternoon: Cup of angelica tea

Late afternoon (or as soon as you return home from work): 15 minute quiet time; read dinner menu

Early evening: Prepare and eat dinner

8.00–9.00: One hour health workshop – Meditation and Contemplation

9.45: Quiet time; review of the day

10.00: To bed

STEP BY STEP

6.00am

As soon as you are properly awake and have written up your dream diary – but before getting out of bed – repeat the affirmation you formulated last night twenty times. Then, when you are ready, stand up and take three slow deep breaths in and out. Relax for a moment, then go through the following stretching sequence (like yesterday morning):

1 Stand relaxed, feet slightly apart. Put your hands together palm to palm in front of you, then stretch your arms up over your head (hands still together). Keeping your arms over your head, stretch the muscles on the right side of your body by bending slowly sideways to the left. Then stretch your left side by bending sideways to the right. Let your arms hang down by your sides and relax.

2 Fold your hands behind your back, fingers interlocked, and stretch your arms downwards and away from your back while you lift your chest forwards and up, arching your spine and looking upwards and backwards as far as you can. Then let your hands go, straighten your back and neck, look ahead and relax.

3 Stand with your arms by your sides, feet a little apart. Lower your head very slowly forward until your chin touches your chest, then continue to bend forwards, curving your back slowly and progressively from the top downwards (keeping your lower back straight as long as possible). Your head and arms should hang down loose and heavy as you bend. When your fingertips are at the same level as your knees, unfold yourself by uncurling your back from the bottom upwards, breathing deeply and sighing as you breathe out. Stand upright and relax.

4 Hold your hands up in front of your heart, palms together. As you take a slow deep breath in, lift your arms upwards as far as you can reach, palms still together. As you breathe out, move your hands apart, outwards and backwards in a big circle, ending up with your palms meeting in front of your heart again. Stand still for a moment, breathing gently.

Now make yourself a cup of angelica tea: 1 tsp of dried herb to a cup of boiling water, brew for a minute or two, strain if necessary. Angelica is quite bitter, so don't make the tea too strong. After your tea, use the bathroom and have a warm bath or shower. If you are having a bath, add 3 drops of frankincense essential oil mixed with 1 tsp sweet almond oil to the water. If you prefer a shower, dilute 3 drops of frankincense oil in 2 tsp sweet almond oil and rub it into your skin after your shower.

6.30am

When you are washed and dressed, go into your quiet space, light a candle and repeat your affirmation twenty times before sitting quietly for five minutes, letting your mind wander where it will. Then read the following Thought for the Day.

Thought for the Day

Whatever you can do, or dream you can, begin it! Boldness has genius, magic and power in it.

GOETHE

φ

Now lie down and go through the simple relaxation exercise you used on Day 6, i.e., think about each part of your body in turn – starting at the feet and working up through legs, bottom, back, arms, shoulders, neck and face – letting each part feel as heavy as possible, as if sinking into the floor. Lie still for a minute without thinking about anything in particular, then repeat the exercise.

Get up, have a good stretch and a yawn, and look briefly through the rest of this Daily Programme Guide, concentrating on the breakfast and lunch menus. When you have collected your thoughts, leave your quiet space and make breakfast.

7.00–8.00am Breakfast (plus prepare lunch if necessary)

Breakfast Menu 1 glass unsweetened fruit juice or spring water • muesli with fruit, nuts and seeds.

You will need (per person):

1 portion sugar-free muesli base

2 tbs mixed chopped nuts/seeds (e.g. walnuts, hazelnuts, almonds, pine
    kernels, sunflower seeds, sesame seeds)

2 dates, chopped

2 dried apricots, chopped

5 tbs mixed fresh fruit/berries, chopped

Mix the muesli base with the nuts and dried fruits, sprinkle the fresh fruit on top and serve with soya milk to taste.

❧ **Health Notes**

Vitamins are substances vital for normal health but which are needed only in small amounts. Some vitamins are made by the body itself – for example, vitamin B3 and vitamin D – and some are synthesized by bacteria that live in our intestines (vitamin K, biotin, pantothenic acid and vitamin B12). Most are obtained from our food, and plant foods as a group are the most important sources of vitamins in the human diet. They are, in fact, the only reliable source of beta-carotene (vitamin A) and vitamin C, and the main contributors of folic acid, biotin and vitamin K. Here is a short check list of the functions of the different vitamins:

B1 – helps us make use of the energy contained in carbohydrate, fat and alcohol, and protects against beri-beri (a syndrome of muscle weakness, heart failure and nerve problems).

B2 – helps us to release energy from food.

B3 – helps us to release energy from food and protects against pellagra (a syndrome consisting of skin rash, weakness, diarrhoea and mental disturbance.

B6 – necessary for normal protein metabolism, for making haemoglobin and for normal central nervous system function.

B12 – vital for normal growth and development of blood cells and normal function of the nervous system.

Folate – helps maintain healthy skin, hair, sweat glands, nerves and bone marrow and is also important in the metabolism of carbohydrates, fats and proteins and to ensure normal development of the baby's nervous system during pregnancy.

Pantothenate – the 'anti-stress vitamin', necessary for normal function of the immune and nervous systems and helps us to make use of the energy in food.

C – an important antioxidant which helps maintain the health of all body tissues.

A – necessary for normal vision and healthy skin; also an important antioxidant.

D – helps us to absorb calcium from our food and protects against rickets and osteomalacia.

E – an important antioxidant necessary for normal red blood cell function.

K – necessary for normal blood clotting, and may help prevent osteoporosis.

Mid-Morning break

A cup of angelica tea. If you feel hungry, have some fresh or dried fruit. If you have time, use some of your break to repeat your affirmation.

Lunchtime

Lunch Menu Catalan salad • fresh fruit

> *You will need (per person):*
> 1 portion lettuce leaves, shredded
> green beans, left over from yesterday, chopped
> potatoes, left over from yesterday, chopped
> 1 tb sweetcorn
> 1 spring onion, chopped
> piece of bread
> 1tbs capers

Put the lettuce leaves on a large plate and arrange the rest of the ingredients on top. Serve with French dressing and a piece of bread.

If you feel like it, have 1 thick slice of pineapple for dessert.

⋙   Health Notes

Minerals and trace elements perform many important functions in the body. They help to build and maintain healthy bones, allow vitamins to function properly, and work with enzymes and other chemicals involved in metabolism. They also play a part in keeping blood and body fluids at the right concentration. You can obtain all the minerals you need to be healthy from food, and many fruits and vegetables contain minerals ready-packaged with other nutrients that make them easier to absorb. Parsley, for example, contains iron and also vitamin C, which makes the iron easier to absorb. Here is a short checklist of the functions of some important minerals:

Calcium – necessary for healthy bones, muscles and teeth, and as a component of various enzymes and hormones.
Magnesium – helps us to make use of the energy stored in our tissues, and is necessary for the efficient use of B-vitamins and calcium by the body.
Iron – used to make haemoglobin (the chemical that enables red blood cells to carry oxygen around the body), enzymes, hormones and bile.

Potassium – necessary for normal cell function, especially nerves and heart muscle.

Zinc – used in the making of carbohydrate and insulin, and is necessary for normal wound healing and normal prostate function.

Selenium – important antioxidant, helps protect against cancer, heart disease and infertility.

Copper – necessary for normal blood cells and bones, and for a healthy nervous system.

Manganese – necessary for normal bones and for normal protein, fat and cholesterol metabolism.

Molybdenum – necessary for normal fat and protein metabolism and may help protect against cancer and tooth decay.

Chromium – necessary for normal blood sugar control.

After lunch, sit quietly for five minutes before taking your midday walk. As you walk, take the chance to repeat your affirmation.

Mid-afternoon break

A cup of angelica tea. If you feel hungry, have some fresh or dried fruit. If you have time, use some of your break to repeat your affirmation.

Late afternoon (or as soon as you return home from work)

Spend fifteen minutes in your quiet space, sitting or lying down quietly. Take a glass of water, unsweetened fruit juice or vegetable juice with you if you feel thirsty. Before leaving your quiet space, read through the dinner recipes below.

Dinnertime

Dinner Menu Stuffed mushrooms with rice, and creamed spinach

You will need (per person):

For the stuffed mushrooms:
100g/4oz brown rice
3–4 large flat open mushrooms

1 tbs olive oil

½ tsp thyme

1 clove garlic

1 tsp soya sauce

2 tbs breadcrumbs

1 tbs fresh parsley, chopped

Rinse the rice well and put in a saucepan with twice the volume of water (plus ¼tsp salt to taste). Bring to the boil then simmer very gently until the water is just absorbed (30–40 minutes). Remove from the heat and leave to stand for 5 minutes before serving. **Set aside half the cooked rice to keep in the fridge for use tomorrow.**

While the rice is cooking, clean the mushrooms and cut off the ends of the stalks. Remove the stalks from the caps and place the caps upside down in a greased oven-proof dish or baking tray. Finely chop the garlic and the mushroom stalks and stir-fry them in olive oil for a minute. Add the thyme and the soya sauce and cook for a few more minutes, until the mushroom stalks give off their moisture. Add the breadcrumbs and stir until the liquid is soaked up. Remove from the heat and add the chopped parsley. Fill the mushroom caps with the mixture. When the rice is nearly done, bake the stuffed mushrooms for about ten minutes at 200°C/400°F/gas mark 6.

For the creamed spinach:

125g/5oz fresh spinach, chopped (or 100g/4oz frozen spinach)

½ tsp basil

1 tbs olive oil

1 tbs flour

4–5 tbs soya milk

Salt and pepper to taste

Put the spinach in a saucepan and cook in a little water until soft (with fresh spinach, the water left on the leaves after washing them is usually enough to cook them in). Put the oil and flour in a cup and mix to a paste. Add the basil and soya milk to the spinach, heat through and then add the oil and flour mixture little by little, stirring continuously until you have a creamy consistency. Adjust the seasoning and serve with the mushrooms and rice.

⚛ **Health Notes**

We live in an age in which pharmaceutical companies are striving to produce 'a pill for every ill', so it is hardly surprising that neatly packaged tablets containing precise amounts of particular vitamins and minerals have become increasingly popular over the past few years. The problem is that everyone is different in the amount of vitamins and minerals they need each day, and also in the amount of any given vitamin or mineral they absorb from any given meal. What we all share is a remarkable ability to extract exactly what we *need* from our food, as long as our meals contain the necessary nutrients. This is why all nutritionists stress the importance of variety in diet, and also why it is so important to eat as much fresh, unprocessed produce as possible. It is often forgotten that most foodstuffs (and particularly fruits and vegetables) contain a whole variety of vitamins, minerals and trace elements. This means that it is actually very hard to avoid eating enough of the different essential nutrients if we eat a varied plant-centred diet, since the nutrients in one food add to the nutrients of the others. In fact, the beneficial effects of some vitamins and minerals seem to depend on their being eaten as part of a food, not separated out into a tablet.

φ

Sit quietly for a few minutes after your meal before clearing and washing up.

8.00–9.00pm

Health Workshop 8 · MEDITATION

In this workshop you will be exploring meditation, the oldest of all self-healing techniques. As we mentioned on Day 6, people who meditate regularly feel clearer mentally, less tired and more alert, and tend to be less prone to stress-related illness (such as high blood pressure). Since meditation develops the ability to concentrate, it can help to improve performance in all areas of life where good concentration is important. Above all, it makes it possible for us to hear the quiet voice of intuition more clearly.

Before starting the meditation sequence below, try the following short concentration exercise for which you will need five pictures (holiday snaps, pictures taken from a magazine; anything will do), six pieces of paper, a pen, and a clock, watch, stopwatch or kitchen timer which you can use to time sixty seconds.

Place the pictures in a row face down beside you. Take the first one and look at it closely for one minute. Then put it face down again, take the first bit of blank paper and write down everything you can remember about the picture in one minute. Go through the same exercise for each of the five pictures in turn, using separate bits of writing paper for each one. When you have finished writing about the fifth picture, take the first picture and study it closely for a minute again. Put it face down, then take the sixth blank sheet of paper and write down everything you can remember about the picture in one minute. When you have finished, compare the first sheet of paper you wrote with the last one, checking the accuracy of each by looking at the picture.

Meditation Sequence

This sequence consists of four elements: preparation, focusing, guided meditation and contemplation. Go through the different parts one at a time, leaving a short break in between each. Each part should last, between five and ten minutes. Your subconscious will probably act as your internal alarm clock, but you may prefer to set an actual alarm clock so that none of the exercises lasts longer than ten minutes.

Preparation: Make sure that you are wearing loose, comfortable clothes and that the room is warm. You may find it pleasant to have a blanket or shawl wrapped around you. Light a candle or night light, take off your shoes, and sit down in front of the candle on an upright chair with your back straight, lower back touching the seat back, knees bent and feet resting comfortably on the floor – one crossed over the other, back foot just in between the front chair legs. (You could also sit cross-legged on a cushion on the floor, back resting lightly against a wall.) Put your thumb and middle finger tip to tip on each hand, and rest your hands lightly on the top of your thighs. Breathe quietly, mouth slightly open. Let your eyelids fall nearly closed, and focus your attention on a point mid-way between your eyebrows. Sit quietly like this for a time, letting thoughts drift in and out without paying them any attention. Someone once said that thoughts are just waves on the ocean of reality. Watch them form, roll into the shoreline, break and merge once again with the receding waves. Let your thoughts subside in a natural way, neither forcing them out nor firing them up into activity. If you feel a thought 'taking hold', or feel yourself drifting into sleep, use your will-power to keep your attention focused in between your eyebrows. If you feel distracted by a bodily sensation such as an itchy nose, let it subside of its own accord rather than react to it.

φ

Focusing: After a short break for a wriggle, stretch and scratch, sit quietly again in the meditation position, eyelids relaxed and nearly closed, and let your attention rest in turn for a few seconds on different parts of your body in the following sequence: Between the eyebrows ▶ right foot ▶ left hand ▶ top of head ▶ bottom of spine ▶ centre of chest ▶ navel ▶ back of neck ▶ right hand ▶ left foot ▶ between the eyebrows. Try this a few times until you find it easy to shift your full attention from place to place at will.

φ

Guided meditation: Sitting quiet and relaxed in the meditation position, let your eyelids fall nearly closed and imagine yourself entirely surrounded by a circle of shimmering golden light. Focus your attention into your right hand. Bring your right hand up to your chest and place the palm flat over your heart. As you feel the spreading warmth of your hand, transfer your attention to the centre of your chest until you are focused entirely on your heart. Let your hand rest back on your thigh. As you continue to concentrate on your heart, feel it slowly opening like the petals of a flower in the morning sun, revealing at its centre a small bright flame. Let the gentle light from this flame spread slowly outwards until it fills your whole body and beyond, radiating love into the universe. Rest in this state until the image gently fades. When you are ready, gather up the circle of golden light that surrounds you and put it into your heart for safe keeping before slowly opening your eyes.

φ

Contemplation: Meditation is the process of looking inside yourself with a steady gaze; contemplation is looking at what you found there. Rest your eyes on the candle flame, your mind still and your body relaxed, and reflect quietly for a few minutes on what you have just experienced.

φ

Before leaving this workshop, read through the notes below about today's herb and oil, and then look through the 'Preparing for Tomorrow' section.

Today's Herb · ANGELICA *(Angelica archangelica)*

Angelica is one of the oldest known medicinal herbs. It probably originated in the Nordic countries where it was used to protect against infection and against evil spells and enchantment. With the arrival of Christianity, it became associated with the Archangel Michael and the Annunciation. Legend also has it that, during an epidemic of plague, the herb was revealed by an angel as a cure (hence the name). It was certainly a constituent of 'Four Thieves Vinegar', used by thieves to protect themselves against the plague during their raids on its victims! Though better known nowadays as a flavouring for confectionery and liqueurs, it is a warming and stimulating herbal tonic which encourages self-awareness and self-confidence. It can be used to treat chest infections, rheumatism, and indigestion, and can also be used to bring on menstruation.

Today's Oil · FRANKINCENSE (Boswellia thurifera)

Frankincense – or olibanum as it is sometimes called – has been used as incense in religious ceremonies since ancient Egyptian times, and it was once valued as highly as gold. It has an uplifting quality which encourages concentration, making it a useful aid to meditation, contemplation and prayer. It also has a soothing effect on the mind and emotions, and can be used to relieve anxiety, fear, obsession and stress. The Egyptians used frankincense to fumigate sick rooms and also as an ingredient in cosmetics to rejuvenate ageing skin. Its antiseptic, astringent and anti-inflammatory properties are certainly well documented, and it continues to be used in toiletries designed to preserve a youthful complexion.

φ

PREPARING FOR TOMORROW

Tomorrow you will be using the herb vervain and the essential oil sandalwood. Breakfast will be muesli with fruits, nuts and seeds, lunch a beetroot and apple salad with rice, and dinner stuffed courgettes followed by baked apples with sweet tahini sauce. Set your alarm tonight for 6.00am, or two hours before you leave for work or start your normal daily activities. Day Nine – INSPIRATION will start with a cup of vervain tea, stretching exercises, a bath or shower and morning quiet time (including a short meditation).

9.45–10.00pm

Before going to bed, go into your quiet space and sit quiet and relaxed. Breathe deeply in and out a couple of times, then review the day's events as usual. Read the following passage and spend a few minutes reflecting on its meaning before going to bed. Before you go to sleep, repeat your affirmation twenty times.

> *There is a light that shines*
> *Beyond all things on Earth*
> *Beyond us all, beyond the heavens*
> *Beyond the highest*
> *The very highest heavens.*
> *This is the light that shines in our heart.*

> CHANDOGYA UPANISHAD

Sleep well.

Thursday

INSPIRATION

On the ninth day, your awakening higher nature allows new concepts to enter your mind which inspire and encourage.

SUMMARY
꙳

6.00: Awake; dream diary; stretching; cup of vervain tea; bath or shower

6.30–7.00: Quiet time; read through Daily Programme Guide

7.00–8.00: Prepare and eat breakfast; prepare packed lunch if necessary

Mid-morning: Cup of vervain tea

Lunchtime: Lunch, followed by short walk

Mid-afternoon: Cup of vervain tea

Late afternoon (or as soon as you return home from work): 15 minute quiet time; read dinner menu

Dinnertime: Prepare and eat dinner

8.00–9.00: One hour health workshop – Music and Movement in healing

9.45: Quiet time; review of the day

10.00: To bed

STEP BY STEP

6.00am

Write up your dream diary and when you are ready to get out of bed, stand up and take three slow deep breaths in and out. Relax for a minute, then go through the usual stretching sequence:

1 Stand relaxed, feet slightly apart. Put your hands together palm to palm in front of you, then stretch your arms up over your head (hands still together). Keeping your arms over your head, stretch the muscles on the right side of your body by bending slowly sideways to the left. Then stretch your left side by bending sideways to the right. Let your arms hang down by your sides and relax.

2 Fold your hands behind your back, fingers interlocked, and stretch your arms downwards and away from your back while you lift your chest forwards and up, arching your spine and looking upwards and backwards as far as you can. Then let your hands go, straighten your back and neck, look ahead and relax.

3 Stand with your arms by your sides, feet a little apart. Lower your head very slowly forward until your chin touches your chest, then continue to bend forwards, curving your back slowly and progressively from the top downwards (keeping your lower back straight as long as possible). Your head and arms should hang down loose and heavy as you bend. When your fingertips are at the same level as your knees, unfold yourself by uncurling your back from the bottom upwards, breathing deeply and sighing as you breathe out. Stand upright and relax.

4 Hold your hands up in front of your heart, palms together. As you take a slow deep breath in, lift your arms upwards as far as you can reach, palms still together. As you breathe out, move your hands apart, outwards and backwards in a big circle, ending up with your palms meeting in front of your heart again. Stand still for a moment, breathing gently.

Now make yourself a cup of vervain tea: 1 tsp of dried herb or one teabag to a cup of boiling water, brew for a few minutes, strain if necessary. After your tea, use the bathroom and have a warm bath or shower. If you are having a bath, add five drops of sandalwood essential oil mixed with 1 tsp of sweet almond oil to the water. If you prefer a shower, dilute 5 drops of sandalwood oil in 2 tsp of sweet almond oil and rub it into your skin after your shower.

6.30am

When you are washed and dressed, go into your quiet space, light a candle and sit quietly for five minutes. Then go through the following self-massage sequence (the same one you used on Day 5), removing contact lenses first, if you wear them. Massage oil is not required.

1 Hold your arms out in front of you, let your hands hang down loose and shake your wrists gently.

2 Holding your arms still, waggle your hands up and down a few times.

3 Rub your hands together, squeezing each hand with the other and rubbing and squeezing your palms and fingers.

4 Hold your hands up in front of your heart, palms and fingers touching. Press one hand against the other for a few seconds, then relax.

5 Keep your fingers touching, but move your palms apart. Press your fingers together for a few seconds, then relax.

6 Rub your palms together and then lightly run them up over your face and down the back of your head several times in a gentle, flowing movement.

7 Cover your face with your hands and run them firmly downwards and outwards over your cheeks and jaw, then around your neck until your fingers meet at the back.

8 Place your thumbs in the corners of your eyes, just by the bridge of your nose. Press upwards lightly and move your thumbs outwards (following the bony ridge above your eye socket) while your forefingers follow the shape of your eyebrows. Repeat.

9 Place your middle fingers underneath your eyes in the inner corners. Press lightly and move your fingers outwards along the bony ridge below your eye socket. Repeat.

10 Place your middle fingers at the inner corner of your eyes again and, applying gentle pressure, glide them downwards and outwards following the contour of your cheek bones and ending up over your jaw muscles. Repeat.

11 Hold your fingers over your jaw muscles and massage them gently for a few seconds using a circular motion.

12 Let your fingertips meet in the middle of your forehead, just above your nose, palms facing inwards. Press your forehead firmly but gently with your fingertips for a few seconds, and then release. Move your fingers upwards a little, press again then release. Continue like this, moving upwards little by little, following the midline of your scalp right over the top of your head and down the back of your neck.

13 Put your fingertips together again on top of your head, just above the hairline. Press your scalp firmly but gently for a few seconds, then release. Move your fingertips gradually apart and downwards, pressing and releasing, continuing like this until you reach your ears.

14 Put your fingertips on the top of your head again, but now with your hands a couple of inches apart. Work your way backwards, pressing and releasing, ending up on the back of your neck just behind your ears.

15 Rub the palms of your hands together and move them up over your face, over the top of your head, down the back of your neck. Relax.

Now sit down in the meditation position, take a slow deep breath in and, on the out breath, sing a gentle, low pitched *ahhh* sound. Let your eyelids fall nearly closed, and imagine yourself surrounded by a circle of golden light. Focus your attention on a point mid-way between your eyebrows and sit quietly like this for a time, letting thoughts drift by until your mind is peaceful and your body still. After a few minutes, gather the circle of light into your heart, open your eyes and rest your gaze on the candle flame for a minute or two.

Get up, have a stretch and a yawn, and then read through the following Thought for the Day.

Thought for the Day

If you have built castles in the air, your work need not be lost. That is where they should be. Now put foundations under them.

HENRY DAVID THOREAU

φ

Look briefly through the rest of this Daily Programme Guide, concentrating on the breakfast and lunch menus. When you have collected your thoughts, leave your quiet space and make breakfast.

7.00–8.00am: Breakfast (plus prepare lunch if necessary)

Breakfast Menu   1 glass unsweetened fruit juice or spring water • muesli with fruit, nuts and seeds

You will need (per person):
1 portion sugar-free muesli base
2 tbs mixed chopped nuts/seeds (e.g. walnuts, hazelnuts, almonds, pine kernels, sunflower seeds, sesame seeds)
2 dates, chopped
2 dried apricots, chopped
5 tbs mixed fresh fruit/berries, chopped
Soya milk

Mix the muesli base with the nuts and dried fruits, sprinkle the fresh fruit on top and serve with soya milk to taste.

☘ Health Notes

Although they have become a part of modern daily life, artificial additives would be entirely unnecessary if we all decided to eat fresh, unprocessed food. The food-processing industry has the right to maximize profit, but we as individuals have the right to expect that those we pay to produce our food will provide us with high quality, unadulterated, safe produce. To give up this right would be to give up our natural heritage of good health, and sadly the evidence is that the rise of 'diseases of civilisation' such as heart disease, stroke and cancer has mirrored the increasing adulteration of our food. Some food additives – vitamin C and lecithin, for example – occur in nature, but the following are all associated with adverse effects on health and should therefore be avoided whenever possible: E102, E104, E107, E110, E122, E123, E124, E127, E128, E131, E132, E133, E142, E150, E151, E154, E155, E160b, E180, E210–219, E220–27, E249–252, E310–312, E320, E321, E407, E413, E416, E450, F466, E620–623, E627, E631, E924, saccharin and aspartame.

Mid-morning break

A cup of vervain tea. If you feel hungry, have some fresh or dried fruit.

Lunchtime

Lunch Menu   Beetroot and apple salad • Rice salad

You will need (per person):

For the beetroot and apple salad:
1 medium-sized raw beetroot, grated
1 sweet apple, grated
1 tbs fresh mint, chopped
juice of 1 orange
¼ tsp cinnamon

Mix the beetroot, apple and mint together in a bowl, pour over the orange juice and sprinkle with cinammon.

> **For the rice salad:**
> **Half** of the cooked rice left over from yesterday. **Save the other half for this evening's recipe.**
> 6 cauliflower florets
> 1 small carrot, finely chopped
> 3 radishes, chopped
> ½ avocado, chopped
> 1 tbs fresh chopped chives

Mix the rice with the cauliflower, carrot, radishes and avocado in another bowl and sprinkle with chives. Season to taste. Serve with the beetroot and apple salad.

✼ Health Notes

Salt – sodium chloride – is a vital component of our blood and body fluids, and conditions that cause us to lose salt from the body put us at risk of life-threatening dehydration. The average Westerner now consumes more that twenty times the amount of salt actually needed for health. High salt intake is associated with high blood pressure – a major risk factor for heart attack and stroke – and it has been estimated that cutting the average salt intake of the population would save tens of thousands of lives each year. Contrary to what many people believe, most salt in our diet comes from food itself, not from added table salt. Since fresh, unprocessed foods contain very much less salt than processed foods, and since most plant-based foods contain much less salt than animal-based foods, the simplest way to cut down on salt is to eat more fresh, unprocessed plant-based foods and reduce the consumption of processed, animal-based produce.

φ

After lunch, sit quietly for five minutes before taking your midday walk. As you walk, try this simple observation exercise: listen to the sounds around you and notice which ones predominate.

Mid-afternoon break

A cup of vervain tea. If you feel hungry, have some fresh or dried fruit.

Late afternoon (or as soon as you return home from work)

Spend fifteen minutes in your quiet space, sitting or lying down quietly. Take a glass of water, unsweetened fruit juice or vegetable juice with you if you feel thirsty. Before leaving your quiet space, read through the dinner recipe below.

Dinnertime

Dinner Menu   Stuffed courgette with steamed vegetables
• Baked apple with sweet tahini sauce

> *You will need (per person):*
>
> **For the stuffed courgette:**
> 1 large courgette
> 2 tbs olive oil
> 1 clove garlic, chopped
> 1 shallot (or ½ onion), finely chopped
> rice (remaining half left over from yesterday)
> 2 mushrooms, chopped
> 25g/1oz spinach (or other greens), finely chopped
> 1 tbs soya milk
> ½ tsp oregano
> salt and pepper to taste

Clean the courgette and cut off the end. Halve it lengthwise and make two hollow 'boats' by scooping out some of the flesh. Place in a greased oven-proof dish, and pre-heat the oven to 200°C/400°F/gas mark 6. Heat the oil gently in a pan, add the garlic, onion, mushrooms and spinach and stir-fry for a few minutes. Add the rice, soya milk and herbs and stir well. Remove from the heat, season to taste and fill the courgette boats with the mixture. Bake for 15–20 minutes, and serve with steamed broccoli and steamed carrots.

For the baked apple dessert:
1 apple
2–3 dates, chopped
1 banana, mashed
1 tbs mixed unsalted nuts, chopped
1 tbs tahini
1 tbs lemon juice
2 tbs maple syrup

While the courgettes are cooking, core the apple and cut a line in the skin horizontally around the middle. Mix half the mashed banana with the chopped dates and stuff the mixture into the apple. Sprinkle the nuts on top. When the courgettes are done, reduce the temperature of the oven to 180°F/350°F/gas mark 4, and bake the apple for about twenty minutes. Just before serving, mix the tahini with the rest of the banana, lemon juice and maple syrup. Add a little water and stir until you have a rich sauce to pour over the baked apple.

⇛ Health Notes

There are many different types of sugar, and the carbohydrate family (of which sugars are a part) is an essential source of energy in the human diet. Not all sugars are good for health, however. One particular sugar – refined sucrose (ordinary white sugar) – causes tooth decay and obesity when eaten in excess, and is associated with a whole range of other diseases including diabetes, Crohn's disease, candida and breast cancer. Since the average Westerner consumes about thirty kilograms of it per year, refined sugar represents a significant health hazard. If we eat a lot of processed food (and about 70 per cent of all food available these days is processed in one way or another), we are bound to eat a lot of sugar since it is added to so many processed products, particularly those that also contain a lot of fat. If, on the other hand, we eat mainly fresh, unprocessed food, we will naturally cut down our refined sugar consumption. So perhaps the best way to regard sugar is like salt – something to be used in small amounts to add interest and flavour to our diet.

φ

Sit quietly for a few minutes after your meal before clearing and washing up. **Before leaving the kitchen, take a couple of minutes to prepare tomorrow evening's dessert** which has to sit in the fridge for twenty-four hours before serving.

Put 50g/2oz chopped dried apricots in a glass serving dish and pour 5 tbs soya milk over them. Cover the dish with a saucer and leave in the fridge.

8.00–9.00pm

Health Workshop 9 · MUSIC & MOVEMENT

For tonight's workshop you will need something to use as a drum (anything from a child's toy to a cardboard box or empty water bottle will do). Wear loose clothing that enables you to move easily, and go barefoot or wear light, flat shoes, according to the floor surface. Clear as much floor-space as possible before starting.

Musical taste is a highly personal thing, but most people have experienced the power of music to uplift and inspire at some time in their lives. Governed by the same fundamental laws that determine the movements of the planets and the proportions of classical architecture, music is a reflection of universal harmony expressed in sound. It can be heard wherever there is joy, celebration and the desire for change, and its rhythms provide the impulse that motivates people to dance.

The human being is a biological symphony, a mass of simple building blocks put together in sequences that harmonize into a whole much greater than the individual parts. When stress and disease make our body-music discordant, music and rhythm can be used to re-establish internal harmony, and there is good evidence that exposing damaged tissues to musical vibration encourages regeneration and healing. In the same way, the mass of electrical impulses in our brain that we call thought can be soothed and quietened by hearing music that speaks to our hearts.

Unfortunately, the move away from individual music-making to recorded sound that characterizes the 'information age' has cut many people off from music as a healing force. Though we hear music almost everywhere, we rarely get the opportunity to feel it. Luckily, we all possess a perfect instrument for musical healing – the human voice. Whether you have a 'good ear' or not, singing encourages wellness by improving breathing, relaxing tense muscles (particularly in the face and solar plexus), exercising the diaphragm, calming the mind and lightening the heart. As you sing, your chest, head, abdomen and spine resonate to the vibrations of the different notes, encouraging the free flow of vital energy which is the foundation of good health. Singing can also provide a way of deepening the experience of meditation, and is a powerful medium of expression for personal prayer and worship.

This workshop is divided into three parts: first, a warm up sequence to help you find your voice; second, a short exercise in rhythm and chanting; and third, a simple musical meditation, incorporating some elements of sacred dance.

WARM-UP

Lie down, open your mouth a little, close your eyes and take a slow gentle deep breath in, then relax and let it out. Feel your diaphragm moving downwards inside you as you suck air in, and up into your chest as you let air out.

Stand up, arms hanging loosely by your sides and take three slow, deep breaths in and out. Count up to nine in your head as you breath in, and back down to one again as you breath out. Concentrate on the smooth movement of your diaphragm (remember, stomach out as you breathe in, stomach in as you breathe out) and remember to keep your shoulders still and relaxed.

Roll your head around slowly, first anti-clockwise then clockwise, to loosen your neck muscles. Then open your mouth as wide as possible, moving your lower jaw around to relax your jaw muscles. With your mouth still open, push your lips as far forward as they will go, then draw them back over your teeth to loosen up your lip muscles. Repeat this three or four times, then relax.

Open your mouth wide, lips pushed a little forward. Take a deep breath in to a count of three and, as you breathe out, make a quiet, sighing *ahhh* sound which falls downwards in pitch until it can go no lower and disappears into the sound of your breath. Repeat this three or four times, making sure that your mouth stays fully open and that your shoulders remain still and relaxed. Stand quietly for a minute.

Open your mouth wide again, lips pushed a little forward, take a deep breath in to a count of three and then sing a low pitched *ahhh* sound to a count of nine. Let your diaphragm move smoothly in order to make the sound as steady as possible. Remember to keep your mouth open and still, and let the note stop gently, without closing your throat. Try this two or three times. (Remember, if you feel at all light-headed doing these exercises, just sit or lie down and breathe quietly for a couple of minutes before continuing.)

SOUND AND RHYTHM

Take your 'drum' and start to beat out a regular, repeating rhythm. Play whatever comes to mind, as long as it is a repeating pattern. If you are not sure what to play, try saying aloud the following rhythmic pattern. Don't leave any gaps between the lines, and go back to the beginning as soon as you reach the end. The tempo should be quite brisk. Use the rhythm as a basis for your drumming.

Dummm de dum dum
Dummm de dum dum
Dummm de dum dum
Radada de dum dum

Once the rhythm is established, and still drumming, open your mouth, push your lips forward, take a deep breath and sing a long, low pitched, nasal *aww* sound as a droning accompaniment to your drumming, taking breaths as necessary. Carry on like this for as long as you want, varying the volume of the drum and the drone, but keeping the rhythm constant. You will probably find that you come to a natural stopping point after a couple of minutes. Rest for a couple of minutes.

MOVING MEDITATION

In your mind's eye, map out a large circle in the middle of the floor and then walk around it slowly in a clockwise direction, putting one foot in front of the other and keeping your paces absolutely even. Let your upper body relax and let your eyes rest in the middle distance, looking at nothing in particular. Concentrate entirely on keeping your paces even and your body upright. When you get back to the starting point, relax for a moment.

Move round the circle again only this time using the following steps. Left – Right – rest back on the left foot – rest forward on the right foot – Left – Right – Left – rest back on the right foot; and so on in a repeating eight-step pattern. On the resting steps, you stop moving forward and lean your weight backwards or forwards on to the foot indicated (in line dancing, this is called rocking forward and back). The forward steps and the resting steps should take the same amount of time so that you move around the circle in a steady rhythm. Concentrate as before on keeping the movements even and your body straight.

Move around the circle again using the same steps, only this time open your mouth, push your lips forward slightly, take a slow deep breath and sing a slow tune in rhythm with your steps (to the sound *ahhh*) as you move round. You can sing any tune you like – preferably just what comes into your head as long as it is slow, simple and in rhythm with your steps – but if you are unsure about what to sing, try *ahhh*ing 'Auld Lang Syne' slowly. The object is to move slowly and evenly while singing steadily and quietly, which takes a surprising amount of concentration. Remember to keep your eyes focused on nothing in particular. You may find it helpful to half close your eyelids. Now relax for a minute and then try again, completing the circle two or three times in a row. Then sit or lie down, and relax quietly for a few minutes.

φ

Before leaving this workshop, read through the notes below about today's herb and oil, and then look through the 'Preparing for Tomorrow' section.

Today's Herb · VERVAIN *(Verbena officinalis)*

The ancient Egyptians called it Tears of Isis, the Romans the 'Herb of Grace', and the Druids regard it as a sacred herb. Once used to ward off the evil eye and treat epileptic fits, vervain is still highly regarded as a treatment for cramps and spasms and as a soothing remedy for nervous complaints. It is an excellent digestive, and its warming, drying and strengthening qualities can be used to relieve all sorts of 'cold' conditions including asthma and the common cold. Its ability to relax the mind and the body make it an important remedy for all stress-related conditions including migraine, anxiety and depression, and it is also useful during convalescence, helping the body to 'recharge the batteries'.

Today's Oil · SANDALWOOD *(Santalum album)*

The name sandalwood comes from a Sanskrit word and the charac-
teristic woody, spicy, rosy and persistent fragrance of sandalwood
oil has been a part of healing and religious ceremony for thousands
of years. A sweet, cooling, natural antibiotic and antiseptic, it will
soothe dry, itchy skin and help clear chronic infection and inflammations of the chest and genito-urinary system. It can also be used
to relieve spasms and cramps. Its calming influence reduces nervous
and emotional tension and it is said to make meditation easier by
encouraging focus and perseverance.

$$\phi$$

PREPARING FOR TOMORROW

Tomorrow, the final day of *Ten Days To Better Health*, you will
be using the herb oats and the essential oil rose. Breakfast will be
porridge with fruits, nuts and seeds, lunch a red cabbage salad
and fresh green salad with tofu, and dinner a lentil and tofu roast
with steamed green vegetables followed by creamed apricots. Set
your alarm tonight for 6.00am, or two hours before you leave
for work or start your normal daily activities. Day Ten – NEW
BEGINNING will start with a cup of herb tea, breathing and
stretching exercises, a bath or shower followed by hydrotherapy
and morning quiet time including self-massage and a short
meditation.

9.45–10.00pm

Before going to bed, go into your quiet space and sit quiet and
relaxed. Breathe deeply in and out a couple of times, then review
the day's events as usual. Read the following passage and spend a
few minutes reflecting on it before going to bed.

At the edge of the cornfield
A bird will sing with them
In the oneness of their happiness
So they will sing together
In tune with the universal power
In harmony with the one creation of all things
And the bird song
And the people's song of life
Will become One

HOPI

Sleep well.

NEW BEGINNING

On the tenth day, you can look to the future refreshed in body, mind and spirit, and with a new confidence in your self-healing ability.

SUMMARY

※

6.00: Awake; dream diary; breathing exercise; stretching; cup of herb tea; bath or shower; hydrotherapy

6.30–7.00: Quiet time; self-massage; meditation; read through Daily Programme Guide

7.00–8.00: Prepare and eat breakfast; prepare packed lunch if necessary

Mid-morning: Cup of herb tea

Lunchtime: Lunch, followed by short walk

Mid-afternoon: Cup of herb tea

Late afternoon (or as soon as you return home from work): 15 minute quiet time; read dinner menu

Early evening: Prepare and eat dinner

8.00–9.00: One hour health workshop – Ceremony and Ritual

9.45: Quiet time; review of the day

10.00: To bed

STEP BY STEP

6.00am

When you have written up your dream diary and are ready to get out of bed, stand up and take three slow deep breaths in and out. Count up to nine in your head as you breathe in and back down to one as you breathe out. Concentrate on the smooth movement of your diaphragm. Relax for a minute, then go through the usual stretching sequence:

1 Stand relaxed, feet slightly apart. Put your hands together palm to palm in front of you, then stretch your arms up over your head (hands still together). Keeping your arms over your head, stretch the muscles on the right side of your body by bending slowly sideways to the left. Then stretch your left side by bending sideways to the right. Let your arms hang down by your sides and relax.

2 Fold your hands behind your back, fingers interlocked, and stretch your arms downwards and away from your back while you lift your chest forwards and up, arching your spine and looking upwards and backwards as far as you can. Then let your hands go, straighten your back and neck, look ahead and relax.

3 Stand with your arms by your sides, feet a little apart. Lower your head very slowly forward until your chin touches your chest, then continue to bend forwards, curving your back slowly and progressively from the top downwards (keeping your lower back straight for as long as possible). Your head and arms should hang down loose and heavy as you bend. When your fingertips are at the same level as your knees, unfold yourself by uncurling your back from the bottom upwards, breathing deeply and sighing as you breathe out. Stand upright and relax.

4 Hold your hands up in front of your heart, palms together. As you take a slow deep breath in, lift your arms upwards as far as you can reach, palms still together. As you breathe out, move

your hands apart, outwards and backwards in a big circle, ending up with your palms meeting in front of your heart again. Stand still for a moment, breathing gently.

Now make yourself a cup of herb tea using whatever herb you found most pleasant over the past nine days. After your tea, have a warm bath or shower. If you are having a bath, add 3 drops of rose essential oil mixed with 1 tsp of sweet almond oil to the water. If you prefer a shower, dilute 3 drops of rose oil in 2 tsp of sweet almond oil and rub over your body afterwards.

Then fill the sink or a bowl with cold water, stand on a towel, dip your hands in the water and rub it over your body, starting with your face and working downwards bit by bit to your feet. Dry yourself vigorously, then get dressed and go into your quiet space.

6.30am

Light a candle and sit or lie down quietly for five minutes. Then go through the usual self-massage sequence, after removing contact lenses, if you wear them. Massage oil is not required.

1 Hold your arms out in front of you, let your hands hang down loose and shake your wrists gently.

2 Holding your arms still, waggle your hands up and down a few times.

3 Rub your hands together, squeezing each hand with the other and rubbing and squeezing your palms and fingers.

4 Hold your hands up in front of your heart, palms and fingers touching. Press one hand against the other for a few seconds, then relax.

5 Keep your fingers touching, but move your palms apart. Press your fingers together for a few seconds, then relax.

6 Rub your palms together and then lightly run them up over your face and down the back of your head several times in a gentle, flowing movement.

7 Cover your face with your hands and run them firmly downwards and outwards over your cheeks and jaw, then around your neck until your fingers meet at the back.

8 Place your thumbs in the corners of your eyes, just by the bridge of your nose. Press upwards lightly and move your thumbs outwards (following the bony ridge above your eye socket) while your forefingers follow the shape of your eyebrows. Repeat.

9 Place your middle fingers underneath your eyes in the inner corners. Press lightly and move your fingers outwards along the bony ridge below your eye socket. Repeat.

10 Place your middle fingers at the inner corner of your eyes again and, applying gentle pressure, glide them downwards and outwards following the contour of your cheekbones and ending up over your jaw muscles. Repeat.

11 Hold your fingers over your jaw muscles and massage them gently for a few seconds using a circular motion.

12 Let your fingertips meet in the middle of your forehead, just above your nose, palms facing inwards. Press your forehead firmly but gently with your fingertips for a few seconds, and then release. Move your fingers upwards a little, press again then release. Continue like this, moving upwards little by little, following the midline of your scalp right over the top of your head and down the back of your neck.

13 Put your fingertips together again on top of your head, just above the hairline. Press your scalp firmly but gently for a few seconds, then release. Move your fingertips gradually apart and downwards, pressing and releasing, continuing like this until you reach your ears.

14 Put your fingertips on the top of your head again, but now with your hands a couple of inches apart. Work your way backwards, pressing and releasing, ending up on the back of your neck just behind your ears.

15 Rub the palms of your hands together and move them up over your face, over the top of your head, down the back of your neck. Relax.

Now sit down in the meditation position, take a slow deep breath in and, on the out breath, sing a gentle, low pitched *ahhh* sound. Let your eyelids fall nearly closed, and imagine yourself surrounded by a circle of golden light. Focus your attention on your heart and sit quietly for a time, letting thoughts drift by until your mind is peaceful and your body still. After a few minutes, gather the circle of light into your heart, open your eyes and rest your gaze on the candle flame for a minute or two. Get up, have a stretch and a yawn, and then read through the following Thought for the Day.

Thought for the Day

> *Truth is within ourselves; it takes no rise*
> *From outward things, whate'er you may believe.*
> *There is an inmost centre in us all,*
> *Where truth abides in fullness; and around,*
> *Wall upon wall, the gross flesh hems it in,*
> *This perfect, clear perception – which is truth.*
>
> *A baffling and perverting carnal mesh*
> *Binds it, and makes all error: and to know*
> *Rather consists in opening out a way*
> *Whence the imprisoned splendour may escape,*
> *Than in effecting entry for a light*
> *Supposed to be without.*
>
> *Paracelsus*, ROBERT BROWNING

φ

Look briefly through the rest of this Daily Programme Guide, concentrating on the breakfast and lunch menus. When you have collected your thoughts, leave your quiet space and make breakfast.

7.00–8.00am: Breakfast (plus prepare lunch if necessary)

Breakfast Menu 1 glass unsweetened fruit juice or spring water • porridge with fruit and nuts

You will need (per person):

3–4 tbs rolled oats

1 tbs mixed chopped nuts/seeds (e.g. walnuts, hazelnuts, almonds, pine kernels, sunflower seeds, sesame seeds)

1 tbs dried fruit (e.g. raisins, apricots)

water

soya milk

½ apple (grated)

Put the oats in a saucepan with the nuts/seeds and the dried fruit. Add twice the volume of water. Bring to the boil, stirring continuously, then simmer very gently until the oats swell and the porridge thickens. Add a little cold soya milk and stir from time to time to stop the porridge sticking to the bottom of the pan. Serve with a little soya milk, maple syrup and some grated apple.

ᚱ Health Notes

Soya beans are an extremely versatile and valuable food source, rich in protein, calcium, magnesium, zinc, potassium, folate, fibre and polyunsaturated oils. A number of questions have been raised, however, over the presence of substances in soya products that may be detrimental to health (such as phytates, phyto-oestrogens and aluminium). On balance, for adults eating a varied diet, the amounts of these substances in soya products do not constitute a particular health risk, and there is even evidence that phyto-oestrogens may be protective against breast and prostate cancer. The effects of phyto-oestrogens on babies fed soya-milk formula foods are currently under investigation. Levels of aluminium in baby milks of all sorts – and in soya-based products in particular – are also justifiable cause for concern, given the possible (but unproven) link between aluminium and Alzheimer's disease. The recent introduction of pesticide-tolerant, genetically modified soya beans into the human food chain is simply another reason for avoiding processed food products (which often contain soya flour), and for eating organic whenever possible.

Mid-morning break

A cup of herb tea of your choice. If you feel hungry, have some fresh or dried fruit.

Lunchtime

Lunch Menu Red cabbage salad • Fresh green salad with tofu

You will need (per person):

For the red cabbage salad:
50g/2oz red cabbage, finely sliced
50g/2oz cauliflower, cut into small florets
½ apple, cut into small cubes

Mix the cabbage and the cauliflower in a bowl and sprinkle the apple cubes over.

For the fresh green salad with tofu:
1 handful lettuce, shredded
½ endive, sliced
2 tbs mixed nuts, chopped
1 tbs olive oil
50g/2oz smoked tofu, cut into small cubes
1 tbs soy sauce

Mix the lettuce and endive in another bowl and toast the nuts in a dry frying pan over a low heat. When just brown, pour the nuts over the lettuce and endive. Put the oil into the frying pan, add the tofu cubes and fry for a few minutes. Remove from heat, sprinkle soy sauce over then add to the lettuce, endive and nuts. Serve both salads with French dressing to taste, and a slice of bread.

⚛ Health Notes

There is no doubt that a good intake of calcium from our diet is important. It provides structure and strength to teeth and bones, helps our heart, muscles and nerves to work efficiently; and forms part of many enzymes and hormones. The commonly held belief that cow's milk is the best dietary source of calcium is simply untrue, and the persistence of the idea owes more to marketing than to science. There is no need to drink milk, eat cheese or take supplements to get enough calcium. It is found in many different plant foods and a plant-centred diet is bound to be rich in calcium. Spring greens, spinach, watercress, parsley, nuts, seeds, seaweed, dried apricots and soya products are just some of the good plant sources of calcium, and gram for gram tofu contains four times more calcium than whole cow's milk. When it comes to avoiding osteoporosis, obtaining calcium from fruits and vegetables may be particularly beneficial since they contain boron, a chemical which helps us to retain calcium in our bodies and which also raises blood oestrogen levels.

φ

After lunch, sit quietly for five minutes before taking your midday walk. As you walk, look around you and notice how many people are smiling.

Mid-afternoon break

A cup of herb tea of your choice. If you feel hungry, have some fresh or dried fruit.

Late afternoon (or as soon as you return home from work)

Spend fifteen minutes in your quiet space, sitting or lying down quietly. Take a glass of water, unsweetened fruit juice or vegetable juice with you if you feel thirsty. Before leaving your quiet space, read through the dinner recipe below.

Dinnertime

Dinner Menu   Lentil and tofu roast • Creamed apricots
(prepared last night)

> *You will need (per person):*
> 50g/2oz red lentils
> 1 shallot (or ½ medium onion), chopped
> ½ clove garlic, chopped
> 1 tbs olive oil
> ½ tsp curry powder (optional)
> ½ teaspoon coriander seeds
> small pinch cayenne pepper (optional)
> 4 tbs vegetable stock
> 1 tsp fresh basil (or ½ tsp dried)
> 50g/2oz tofu, crumbled
> salt and pepper to taste

Check the lentils for small stones, rinse well under running water and place in a saucepan with double their volume of water. Bring to the boil, skim off any froth and simmer gently until soft (about 15 minutes), adding a little more water from time to time if necessary. While the lentils are cooking, pre-heat the oven to 200°C/ 400°F/gas Mark 6. Heat the oil in a frying pan, add the spices, shallot and garlic and stir-fry gently for a few minutes. Add the 4 tbs water/vegetable stock, heat through and pour into a mixing bowl together with the cooked lentils. Add the basil and the tofu, mix well and season to taste. Pour the mixture into a greased ovenproof dish and bake for 45 minutes. Serve with a mixed salad or steamed green vegetables. (This dish also tastes good cold.)

🌿 Health Notes

More and more people are reducing their consumption of dairy products because, despite its homely reputation, cow's milk compromises health in four ways. 1. It can provoke asthma, hay fever and eczema in those allergic to it. 2. It is high in saturated and trans fats and is thus a risk factor for heart disease. 3. It is often contaminated with hormones, antibiotics and other agrochemical residues which may produce unpredictable adverse reactions. 4. It contains a sugar – lactose – which we lose the ability to digest efficiently after about the age of five. What is more, many people with catarrhal problems, candida and arthritis experience substantial relief when they exclude dairy products from their diet, although the reasons for this are not clear. No other species routinely consumes large quantities of the breast milk of another species, a substance which is designed to feed babies. It is time we weaned ourselves off milk and on to a fresh, plant-centred diet – supplemented according to taste and conscience with some fresh, humanely reared and slaughtered meat and fish. We have nothing to lose but our ill health.

φ

Sit quietly for a few minutes after your meal before clearing and washing up.

8.00–9.00 pm

Health Workshop 10 · CEREMONY & RITUAL

This workshop marks the end of *Ten Days To Better Health*. We hope you have experienced some new feelings and sensations, new tastes and new understandings, and that you have a heightened awareness of your body. We also hope that you have learned some techniques that make you feel good in yourself and about yourself, and that you feel better and brighter than when you began.

Before starting, read through the notes below about today's herb and oil.

Today's Herb · OATS *(Avena sativa)*

Oat is an ancient plant with a long history of use as both food and medicine. As well as providing a solid and reassuring start to the day as a breakfast food in porridge and muesli, oats can be used to soothe digestive disturbances, ease stress and and give new energy to a tired nervous system. The non-starch polysaccharide (fibre) in oats helps to lower blood cholesterol and fat levels and thus reduces the risk of coronary heart disease.

Today's Oil · ROSE *(Rosa damascena and centifolia)*

The rose, queen of flowers, is a timeless symbol of love and devotion. The essential oil has cooling, calming, cleansing and toning qualities which make it an excellent antidote to stress, and a useful remedy for inflammations and swellings. It can be used also to ease problems relating to the female reproductive system, and is soothing and healing to dry skin. Above all, rose has the ability to increase vitality and wellbeing and, as the flower of the heart, it brings self-confidence, tolerance and understanding to those that use its fragrance.

φ

Ceremony and ritual are natural and important parts of human behaviour, used in all societies to mark ends and beginnings and to ease the transitions of life. They perform a function in society like the subconscious mind performs for the individual since they enable us to act appropriately at important and difficult moments without having to think about what to do. They also provide a vehicle for religious experience by creating an environment which allows us to hear the inner voice of intuition more clearly. People from many different philosophical traditions have discovered that ritual can calm the mind, still the emotions and keep the body occupied, thus allowing a sense of the spiritual or higher self to emerge more clearly.

The elements of ceremony are as follows:

- An introduction, providing the chance to settle down and focus on the present.

- A statement of purpose, setting out the meaning of the ceremony.

- A moment of transition, often silent.

- A moment of transformation, the heart of the ceremony where a promise is made, a vow is taken, or a decision is confirmed which defines the difference between what has gone before and what is to come after.

- A moment of meditation, to reflect on the impact of the change.

- A moment of celebration that a change has been made.

- A moment of completion when the ceremony is ended and a parting thought or statement is spoken.

In summary, ceremony consists of introduction, statement of purpose, transition, transformation, meditation, celebration and completion.

In addition to these basic elements, ceremony can involve the use of visual and other aids to create a sense of occasion. Beautiful clothes and colours, a pleasing environment, nice smells, inspiring music, uplifting poetry and atmospheric lighting can all add to the impact.

In this final workshop, therefore, we invite you to devise and perform a short ceremony for yourself, using the above elements, to mark the beginning of a new phase in your life. It should have two main objectives: to celebrate ten days of change and to confirm your commitment to better health.

Arrange your quiet space in a way you find pleasing, perhaps using a mixture of your favourite essential oils to perfume the air. Have something beautiful arranged on a table in front of you so that you have something to rest your eyes on as the ceremony progresses. If you have a tape-recorder, you could also use music to help create a good atmosphere. You don't have to use many words – all that matters is that they are your words and that you mean what you say. It's not the length of a ritual that counts, it's the clarity. You can speak aloud, speak inside your head, or do both.

Once you have worked out what words you are going to use and have arranged the room and collected your other bits and pieces (oils, candles, tape-recorder and tapes, etc.), take a quick bath or shower and put on some comfortable clothes that make you feel good, or which have good associations for you. Then return to your quiet space, light a candle (or candles) and perform your ceremony.

When you have finished, sit quiet and relaxed for a few minutes. Breathe deeply in and out a couple of times, then review the day's events. Finally, read the following passage aloud before blowing out your candle and going to bed. Thank you for the effort you have put in over the past ten days, and every good wish for the future. May your life be blessed with health, love, peace and light.

> *There will be happiness before us*
> *There will be happiness behind us*
> *There will be happiness above us*
> *There will be happiness below us*
> *There will be happiness around us*
> *And words of happiness shall extend from our mouths*
> *For we are the essence of life*

Goodnight.

CONCLUSION

Now you have finished *Ten Days To Better Health*, take some time to look back over your experiences. Whatever your impressions of the programme, you will have changed by following it and you will have made the first step towards better health. You have probably found that some of the methods used appealed to you more than others. We hope you will feel inspired to carry on with your favourites and include them in your daily routine as part of a new, healthier way of living. Similarly, if you have found that naturopathic nutrition suits your taste, you could incorporate some of the recipes and general principles into your normal diet.

If you do decide to continue using the techniques you have learned, remember that it is better to do stretching, breathing exercises and hydrotherapy before eating, and that meditation is also more effective on an empty stomach (and often easier to do after some physical activity). Relaxation sequences, self-massage and autosuggestion can be practised in spare moments at any time of the day, but musical meditation and ceremony need more time, and are more effective when not constrained by deadlines.

Whether or not you carry on using any of these self-healing methods, you could try and keep some periods of silence, a midday walk and a nightly 'review of the day' in your new rhythm, and include as many fresh, unprocessed fruits and vegetables in your diet as possible. This change alone would greatly reduce the risk of you suffering from serious disease (such as heart disease and cancer) in the future.

You may find it interesting now to fill in the questionnaire on page 172. When you have answered all the questions, look back at the answers you gave ten days ago on page 35, and use the charts on pages 173 and 174 to help you compare how you felt then with how you feel now. If you can see a clear improvement in your general health and wellbeing, you might consider using the programme on a regular basis (once every three to six months) as a way of maintaining better health and vitality.

We hope very much that you have enjoyed *Ten Days To Better Health*, and that you are noticing real and positive benefit from following the programme. Discovering self-healing is a journey not an event, and the path linking where you start with where you want to be is not always straightforward. But as long as you can feel positive change happening within yourself, and see changes for the better occuring in the pattern of your life, you will reach the destination of health which is the goal of all the healing arts.

Questionnaire

How satisfied are you with the following aspects of your life? Choose a number between 0 and 100, 0 meaning completely unsatisfied, 100 meaning you are completely satisfied:

1. Your diet ☐

2. Your sleep ☐

3. Your level of physical activity ☐

4. The amount of time you get to relax ☐

5. The amount of time you get to yourself ☐

6. The amount of time you spend outdoors ☐

7. Your energy level ☐

8. Your general health ☐

9. Your memory and concentration ☐

10. Your work/regular daily activities ☐

11. How peaceful you feel ☐

12. How happy you are ☐

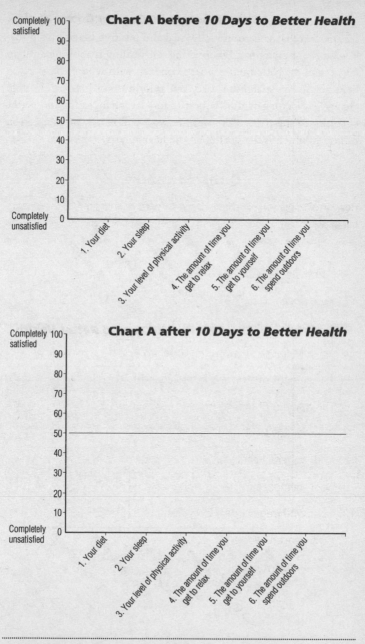

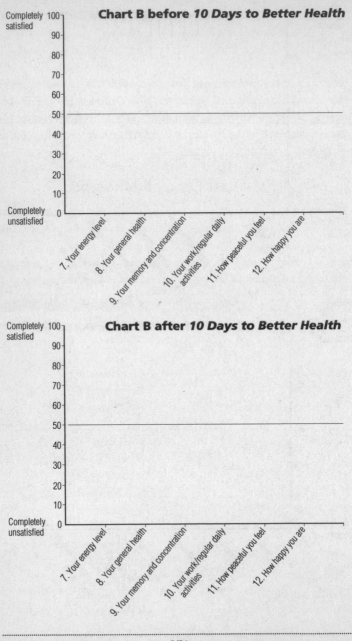

APPENDIX

This appendix contains some further examples of the use of essentail oils, water, fasting and ceremony. You can use them to help you deal with occasional minor ailments, and also to help you regain your balance when the stresses of daily life intrude on your sense of wellbeing.

Essential Oil Combinations

Here are some combinations of essential oils which you can use to help you deal more effectively with the stresses and strains of daily life. For baths, add the essential oils to one teaspoon of sweet almond oil and pour in the bath just before you get in. For massage, dilute the essential oils in two tablespoons of sweet almond oil.

	Essential Oil	No. of drops
Anti-stress	Marjoram	4
	Melissa	1
Exhaustion	Frankincense	1
	Lavender	2
	Rosemary	2
Fear and anxiety	Marjoram	2
	Melissa	1
	Rose	1
	Sandalwood	1
Insect bites (also as insect repellent)	Eucalyptus	2
	Lavender	3
	Melissa	1
Mental fatigue	Frankincense	2
	Rosemary	3

Rejuvenation	Melissa	1
	Frankincense	2
	Rose	1
	Sandalwood	2
Relaxation	Lavender	2
	Rose	1
	Sandalwood	2
Stimulation	Rosemary	2
	Melissa	1
	Frankincense	2

For cuts, sores, and minor skin conditions try the following combination of oils mixed in 2 tablespoons of calendula oil, applied directly but sparingly to the affected area:

Eucalyptus	1 drop
Melissa	1 drop
Sandalwood	1 drop
Lavender	2 drops
Marjoram	2 drops

For sore muscles and joints, add 4 drops each of eucalyptus, marjoram and rosemary to 2 tablespoons olive oil and massage into the affected area.

More Uses of Water

Waist Compress

This simple hydrotherapy technique is designed to encourage inner cleansing and the elimination of accumulated waste via the skin and the kidneys. It can be used to ease pain associated with stomach, kidney, back or period problems, and also to stimulate menstruation and relieve the effects of prostatic enlargement. Since it produces a feeling of deep relaxation, it can be helpful at night to encourage restful sleep.

You will need one piece of thin cotton or linen cloth, 20–25cm wide and long enough to reach all the way around the waist with an overlap. You will also need a strip of warm knitted material, 30cm wide and also long enough to reach around the waist with an overlap. A folded blanket is also suitable.

Lay the knitted material or folded blanket flat along the edge of the bed, and soak the thin material in cold tap water. Wring it out until it no longer drips, then lay the damp cloth on top of the knitted material/folded blanket. Bare your skin from waist to bottom, stand with your back to the compress materials, pick up both layers together and wrap them around your waist in a quick, single movement. Tighten the ends around your front (the quicker you tighten it, the less chilly it feels) and fasten with a couple of safety pins. The wrap should be tight enough to stay in place but without causing any feeling of constriction.

Get into bed and relax for an hour. When you remove the compress, wash the area that was covered in clean warm water and dry thoroughly with a towel. (Be sure to wash the compress materials in hot soapy water before using again.)

After the first mild shock of the cold application, the compress starts to warm up and should feel quite cosy after about five minutes. If it doesn't warm up, the damp cloth may not have been wrung out sufficiently so remove the compress, wait half an hour and start again with a less damp inner cloth. If the second application doesn't warm up in five minutes, remove the compress and don't re-apply. Try one of the other hydrotherapy techniques instead.

Note that using a waist compress may cause slight redness around the waist which will disappear of it own accord. Your urine may also get a little darker – and perhaps stonger smelling – the next day, but this is just a sign that your kidneys are eliminating waste material.

Steam Inhalation

Steam inhalations can be used to relieve sinus and chest conditions and have a clearing and cleansing effect on the head and the airways.

Fill a saucepan with boiling water, bring to the boil and add two tablespoons of dried thyme. Put the lid on the pan, turn off the heat and leave to stand for five minutes.

Put two chairs facing each other, place the pan on one and yourself on the other, wrap a blanket around you and put a big towel over your head. Take the lid off the pan and gently inhale the steam for about ten minutes. Afterwards, splash your face with cool water, then lie down and relax for 15 minutes.

Sitz Bath

Sitz baths are calming and relaxing and are best taken just before bedtime. They can also be used to ease conditions of the kidney and bladder, and to relieve constipation. You can use the bath or a wash-tub.

Pour some cool tap water into the bath or wash tub to a depth of about 15cms. Wrap your shoulders in a blanket and sit in the water until the initial sensation of cold is replaced by a feeling of spreading warmth. This may happen quickly or take a few minutes, depending on your constitution and the temperature of the water. Stand up, dry yourself vigorously, put on pyjamas or a track-suit and relax in bed for at least an hour (or all night if the sitz bath is taken last thing).

Three Day Fast

Occasional fasting is a powerful way of clearing the body of accumulated waste and of reducing susceptibility to illness and the effects of stress. It is particularly effective during the spring and summer, and helps the body to use all available resources for healing and repair. Though short fasts are completely safe for normally healthy people, they should be avoided during pregnancy and breast feeding, and after operations or serious accidents. They are not recommended for people under the age of eighteen, and should not be used by anyone who is very overweight or who has a history of an eating disorder (such as anorexia nervosa or bulimia). If you are on medication, don't fast without seeking the advice of the practitioner who prescribed it (or, if necessary, a registered naturopath). Smoking and alcohol should be avoided during any fast.

The following 'mono-fruit' fast is simple and gentle and involves cutting out all foods except one fruit for three days. We use grapes for this example, but you can use any fruit that 'agrees with you'. For three days before the fast, you should try and cut down progressively on stimulants (tea, coffee, etc.), sugar, processed food, meat and dairy products. This will make the fast itself more pleasant. When you have finished fasting, make a gradual return to 'normal' eating introducing fruits, vegetables and rice before other foods. Make sure the water you drink is as pure as possible, and remember to drink plenty, and whenever you feel thirsty. You are unlikely to experience any significant healing crisis on such a short fast, but you may feel some nausea and notice that your bowels become looser. Your breath and urine may also smell stronger than normal. Such symptoms pass quickly, however, and you will be left feeling fresher and more energetic after the fast. (Remember – you are always in control. If you feel that the fast really isn't suiting you, you can stop at any time.)

Day One: Eat only grapes – as many as you want, whenever you want – and drink water and grape juice.
Day Two: Drink water and grape juice only.
Day Three: Eat only grapes, and drink water and grape juice.

Dealing with Regrets

Living in the present is an important part of being healthy and learning to let go of the past is a powerful aid to self-healing. Of all memories, it is our regrets and our grudges that have the worst effects on our state of wellbeing, and much modern counselling is directed towards dealing with the unfinished business that creates such feelings. In both Eastern and Western mystery traditions, ceremony is often used to enhance the effects of self-analysis and the following simple ritual is a powerful way of clearing the mind of backward-looking negative thoughts. It can be used at any time, but is particularly useful at times of transition between old and new phases in life (such as New Year, career changes, house moves, etc.).

Write down all the regrets you feel – or the grudges you bear – on separate little pieces of paper. Take a metal container and some matches or a lighter, and set fire to each piece of paper in turn, watching each one crumble into ash before lighting the next.

φ

FURTHER READING

O. Alexandersson, *Living Water* (Bath, UK, Gateway Books, 1994)

Ch'u Ta-Kao, *Tao Te Ching* (London, Unwin Paperbacks, 1982)

E. Coué, *The Practice of Autosuggestion* (available from the Metaphysical Research Group, Archer's Court, Hastings, England TN35 4PG)

S. Curtis, *Essential Oils* (London, Aurum Press Ltd, 1996)

D. Frawley and V. Lad, *The Yoga of Herbs* (Santa Fe, Lotus Press, 1986)

M. Fukuoka, *The One Straw Revolution* (Rodale Press, USA, 1978)

M. Grieve, *A Modern Herbal*, edited by C.F. Leyel (London, Tiger Books International, 1992)

B. Haldbo, *Træd Frem* (Copenhagen, Munksgaard, 1996)

K. Hartvig and N. Rowley, *You Are What You Eat* (London, Piatkus Books, 1996)

D. Hoffmann, *The Holistic Herbal*, 2nd edition (Forres, Scotland, The Findhorn Press, 1988)

M. Jaffrey, *Eastern Vegetarian Cooking* (London, Arrow Books Ltd, 1990)

H. Lamont, *The Gourmet Vegan* (London, Victor Gollancz Ltd, 1988)

H. Lindlahr, *Natural Therapeutics*, Volume II, Practice (Saffron Walden, UK, The C.W. Daniel Company Ltd, 1981)

S. Mills, *The Dictionary of Modern Herbalism*, (Wellingborough, UK, Thorsons, 1985)

S. Radhakrishnan, *The Bagavadgita* (London, Aquarian, 1989)

S. Ray, *Indian Vegetarian Cooking* (London, The Apple Press, 1988)

J. Robbins, *Diet for a New America* (Walpole, New Hampshire, Stillpoint Publishing, 1987)

M. Van Straten and B. Griggs, *Superfoods* (Dorling Kindersley, 1990)

R. Tisserand, *The Art of Aromatherapy*, Revised Edition (Saffron Walden, UK, The C.W. Daniel Company Ltd, 1985)

J. Valnet, *The Practice of Aromatherapy* (Saffron Walden, UK, The C.W. Daniel Company Ltd, 1982)

A. Wakeman and G. Baskerville, *The Vegan Cookbook*, 2nd edition (London, Faber and Faber, 1986)

H. Walden, *The Quick After-Work Summer Vegetarian Cookbook* (London, Piatkus Books, 1996)

J. Young, *Self-Massage* (London, Thorsons, 1992)

J. Young, *Acupressure for Health* (London, Thorsons, 1994)

USEFUL ADDRESSES

HERBS AND ESSENTIAL OILS

Neal's Yard Remedies (Mail Order)
8–10 Ingate Place,
Battersea,
London SW8 3NS
Tel: 020 7489 1686
Customer Service Helpline: 020 7627 1949

INFORMATION ON ORGANIC PRODUCE

Henry Doubleday Research Association
Ryton Organic Gardens,
Coventry CV8 3LG
Tel: 024 7630 3517

The Soil Association
Bristol House,
40–56 Victoria Street,
Bristol BS1 6BY
Tel: 0117 929 0661

GENERAL

United Kingdom

The British Naturopathic Association
Goswell House,
2 Goswell Road,
Somerset BA16 0JG
Tel: 08707 456984

The Food Commission/
The National Food Alliance
5–11 Worship Street,
London EC2 2BH

Movement for Compassionate Living
31 Walton Close,
Ernesford Grange,
Coventry CV3 2LJ

The National Institute of Medical Herbalists
56 Longbrook Street,
Exeter, Devon EX4 6AH
Tel: 01392 426022

BCM Permaculture Association
London WC1N 3XX
Tel: 0845 4581805

Positive News (Planetary Connections)
The Six Bells, Church Street,
Bishop's Castle,
Shropshire SY9 5AA

The Vegan Society
7 Battle Road,
St Leonards on Sea,
East Sussex TN37 7AA

The Vegetarian Society
Parkdale, Dunham Road,
Altrincham,
Cheshire WA14 4QG
Tel: 0161 925 2000

United States of America

The American Association of Naturopathic Physicians
3201 New Mexico Avenue,
NW Suite 350,
Washington DC 20016

The American Herb Association
PO Box 1673
Nevada City CA 95959

The American Naturopathic
Medical Association
PO Box 96273,
Las Vegas NV 89193

The National Association of
Holistic Aromatherapy
4509 Interlake Ave N., #233,
Seattle WA 98103-6773

The Natural Hygiene Society
PO Box 30630,
Tampa FL 33630

Australia

The Australian Traditional
Medicine Society
PO Box 1027,
Meadowbank NSW 2114

The National Herbalists
Association of Australia
13 Breillat Street,
Annandale NSW 2038

Association of Massage Therapists
PO Box 358,
Prahran,
Victoria Australia 3181

New Zealand

South Pacific College of Natural
Therapeutics,
PO Box 11311,
Auckland

Canada

The Ontario Herbalists'
Association
R.R. #1,
Port Burwell, Ontario,
N0J 1T0 Canada

Ontario Association of
Naturopathic Doctors
344 Bloor Street West,
Suite 602,
Toronto
Ontario M5S 3A7

INDEX